psychiatric and mental health nursing: a commitment to care and concern

helen z. kreigh, r.n., b.s.n.ed., m.a.

joanne e. perko, r.n., b.s.n., m.n.ed.

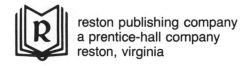

reston publishing company
a prentice-hall company
reston, virginia

Library of Congress Cataloging in Publication Data

Kreigh, Helen Z.
  Psychiatric and mental health nursing.

  Includes bibliographies.
  1. Psychiatric nursing. I. Perko, Joanne E.,
joint author. II. Title. [DNLM: 1. Psychiatric
nursing. WY160.3 K92p]
RC440.K73   610.73'68   79-4463
ISBN 0-8359-5711-X

©1979 by Reston Publishing Company, Inc.
A Prentice-Hall Company
Reston, Virginia 22090

10 9 8 7 6 5 4 3 2

Printed in the United States of America

contents

chapter fourteen–psychopathology: symptoms, dynamics and principles 157

PART THREE 193

chapter fifteen–nursing intervention for patients with thought disorders 195

chapter sixteen–nursing intervention for patients with feeling disorders 205

chapter seventeen–nursing intervention for patients with disturbances in behavior 219

chapter eighteen–nursing intervention for patients experiencing procedure-oriented activity 241

chapter nineteen–planning effective nursing care: rules of thumb ...253

preface

While comparing our separate and diverse backgrounds and years of experience as educators and clinical practitioners in psychiatric-mental health nursing, we discovered that our students and colleagues share a common problem. The problem as we see it relates to their struggle to formulate operational nursing activity from a multiplicity of theories and psychiatric concepts. For example, time after time, we have been approached and asked such questions as: "What do I do when a patient doesn't keep a scheduled appointment?"; "How do I get a patient interested in occupational therapy?"; "When the textbook says to 'motivate the patient,' what exactly does that mean and how do I do it?"; "What do I say to a patient when he tells me he feels hopeless, lonely or that he wants to die?"; and "How do I get the time to do the kinds of things I know are necessary for good patient care?"

It is in response to these questions and others like them that we have undertaken the task of setting down some of the day-to-day aspects, approaches and interventions that we have found useful and effective. It is our hope that from the many suggestions we will present, students entering the field of psychiatric-mental health nursing for the first time will be provided with a starting point—a set of guidelines. In other words, we offer steppingstones from which the beginner can discover and develop the potential therapeutic self.

Although the focus of our attention is geared toward assisting students in developing practice skills, we recognize that some of these same questions are asked by practitioners in various types of patient care settings. For the practitioner, we offer a ready practice reference which supplies concrete, realistic interventions geared to meeting those recurring problems and concerns. For the nurse who is seeking to improve her practice, we believe that the suggestions, approaches and methods will act as the stimulus she needs to spark and rekindle her creativity and imagination.

We have divided our book into four main parts, each part with a particular focus. *Part One* focuses on the nurse, her development and acquisition of the fundamental knowledge, art and skills needed for the practice of psychiatric-mental health nursing. *Part Two* is concerned with the presentation of a theoretical framework regarding man, his development and those adaptive responses which either enhance or hinder his physiological or psychological state of equilibrium. *Part Three* is specifically directed toward the identification of nursing care goals, approaches and interventions which we believe are applicable to any patient experiencing psychological distress, regardless of diagnostic label or practice setting. The focus is on the common, recurring nursing care problems most frequently encountered by practitioners and some of the nursing care measures we have found to be conducive to the effective delivery of nursing care. In *Part Four*, because of our belief as educators that most students require definitive guidelines, and because students in a psychiatric setting rarely encounter the progression of patient care from admission through discharge, we include a case presentation. In this way we are able to show the scope of the nursing intervention process: the identification of pathology or areas of dysfunction; the effects of admission; the assessment process; the utilization of the problem-solving approach; and the way in which nurse-patient interaction is conducted, recorded and evaluated along with the provision for follow-up aftercare.

As educators and practitioners, we feel that learning and knowledge without skillful application results in disservice to patients and reflects a lack of commitment to care and concern for patients as people. Thus, we feel there is a genuine need to emphasize the practical aspects which demonstrate how learning is transferred and how knowledge is applied to the real situations encountered by the nurse in her everyday practice.

For ease of reading, the pronoun "she" is used to refer to the nurse and the pronoun "he" is used to refer to the patient.

acknowledgements

We wish to express our sincere thanks and appreciation to all those who assisted us in making this book a reality. To Mike and the Kreigh kids we thank humbly for their inspiration, cooperation and willingness to do without, understanding our special needs and most of all for their unfailing faith in our ability to succeed. To all our colleagues both in and out of nursing we are grateful for their support, encouragement and the opportunities they provided to clarify our thinking. To our students we extend special thanks for voicing the questions and concerns which triggered our literary effort. We are particularly appreciative of the effort of Frances Ward who contributed ideas for some of the illustrations and who together with Pat Gallagher transcribed our initial scribbling into a readable rough draft. And to Rosemary Scirocco, our friend and colleague, our grateful appreciation for her critical comments, professional expertise, editorial adjustments and unfailing sense of humor. To Richard J. Perko our heartfelt thanks for freely giving of himself to ease the demands of family responsibility, for investing his time, effort and energy throughout, in particular during the final preparation of the manuscript and lastly for his subtle, witty comments which stimulated our efforts.

In loving memory we dedicate this book to our parents:
Mrs. Elsie J. Perko
Mrs. Elmira Kreigh
Mr. Anthony J. Zankofski
Dr. Adolph J. Perko
all who died since the writing of this book was begun.

part 1

a commitment to care and concern

learning objectives

On completion of this chapter the reader should be able to:

1 Define and differentiate between *mental health* and *mental illness.*
2 Recognize the implications mental illness has for an individual and for society.
3 Recognize the implications that an awareness of mental health and mental illness has for the practice of nursing.
4 Define the term *psychiatric-mental health nursing.*
5 Identify the basic philosophy and framework of psychiatric-mental health nursing practice.

mental health—mental illness

In the psychiatric-mental health field, much of the literature points toward the existence of a continuum between mental health and mental illness. This view of health and illness implies linear movement from one extreme of the continuum to the other. At any given time in an individual's life his functioning is reflected by a specific point along the continuum. Where the point lies depends on the individual's ability to satisfy his needs. The position changes as the individual responds and reacts to the impact of his current reality, thereby affecting his functioning. Correspondingly, the statement is made that no one has absolute health or is "completely normal." However, seldom does one hear or see a disavowal of the claim of absolute illness. The individual is either mentally ill or not; that is, the person is identified as having a specific set of symptoms and is therefore labeled as having a specific clinical condition. For us, this way of explaining an individual's ability to cope is not completely satisfactory.

An alternative way of expressing an individual's relationship to himself, to others and to his environment is to state that both health and illness exist on a separate and distinct continuum. Thus, on the health continuum there are specific criteria used in the assessment of variations in mental functioning and in identifying the degree of maturity. On the illness continuum there are specific behaviors which manifest the existence of a pathological process and which are indicative of its severity. In keeping with this viewpoint, when a healthy individual encounters crisis and is temporarily unable to satisfactorily resolve the crisis, he remains a healthy person but moves toward the lower end of the health continuum. If, on the other hand, a healthy individual is subjected to sustained stress or crisis, over a prolonged period of time, he moves from the health continuum to the illness continuum. In the first instance, where the healthy individual moves from one extreme of the health continuum to the other, he remains able to initiate coping devices or learn alternative means of adaptation, usually without therapeutic intervention. This is not so in the second instance, where the individual moves from the health continuum to the illness continuum. This individual will need therapeutic intervention. The goal of therapeutic intervention is to return the individual to optimal functioning along the health continuum.

Mental health is an evolving process in which the individual's internal demands and needs are brought into harmonious relationship with the reality of the environment in which he lives. Its achievement is obtained through successful adaptation. Successful adaptation in daily living requires that an individual establish a point of equilibrium between his wants, needs, abilities, ambitions, values and feelings and the real or perceived expectations of the society and surrounding environmental influences in which the individual operates. Consequently, the individual is able to function independently without distorting reality while gaining mastery over himself and his environment. Thus, a *mentally healthy person* is one who possesses the ability to make adjustments which enable him to remain unhampered by emotional conflict and free from pathological symptomatology; confirm and follow a philosophy of living; find satisfaction and fulfillment in exercising and expanding his potential; and establish and maintain meaningful relationships with others.

Mental illness is a personal as well as a social problem. It is disruption, disorganization, dysfunction or disintegration. As a personal problem, *mental illness* is maladjustment in living. It produces a disharmony in a person's thoughts, feelings and actions. In mental illness, the individual loses his ability to respond according to the expectation he has for himself and the demands that society has for him. In essence, mental illness is a failure on the part of the individual to adapt and vary his responses within the context of his current reality. In mental illness, the individual's reaction to himself, his interactions with others and with his environment are usually inadequate, inappropriate and unacceptable, reflecting the extent of his emotional, psychological and physical dysfunction.

The presence of mental illness and the extent of its influence produces an economical and political threat to society. Economically, mental illness decreases society's productivity through: 1) reducing either the numbers or the efficiency of the labor force, thus affecting the gross national product; and 2) placing budgetary constraints on the general economy because of the need to allocate a substantial amount of available funds toward treatment facilities and programs. Politically, the ramifications of social deviance, non-conformity and the unpredictable nature of mental illness undermines the power structure of society through its psychological impact on all the members of society. Society is not concerned so much with the presence of disability as it is concerned with the presence of deviance which in turn generates increased tension, disruption and fear. Thus, mental illness is a complex problem which in its broadest sense implies an all-encompassing umbrella-like concept used to designate psychological, emotional and social disequilibrium.

characteristic differences between mental health and mental illness

To provide the reader with a clear, concise overview of the major, significant, descriptive elements distinguishing a mentally healthy person from that of a mentally ill person, we have made the following comparisons. These comparisons are based on the relationship that the self maintains toward the self, toward others, and with the environment.

TABLE 1-1
COMPARISON BETWEEN MENTAL HEALTH AND MENTAL ILLNESS

Mental Health	Mental Illness
Relationship With Self	
Possesses self-knowledge and a sense of identity	Self-identity is distorted and not based in reality
Accepts self, both strengths and weaknesses	Unable to accept strengths or weaknesses
Accepts criticism	Rejects and/or denies criticism
Meets or postpones gratification of basic needs	Depends on others to meet basic needs

TABLE 1-1 (continued)

Mental Health	Mental Illness
Relationship With Self	
Sets appropriate short- and long-term goals and moves toward actualization	Inappropriate goal setting with ineffective organization and planning
Establishes a value system	Value system fluctuates indiscriminately
Uses past experience to illuminate the present and to plan for the future	Focuses on the past; has a limited awareness of before-and-after effects
Assumes responsibility for self-learning	Demonstrates limited incentive to learn and is negativistic
Values productivity; achieves satisfaction and enjoyment from work	Uses work to avoid involvement and responsibility in the growth process; work is nonproductive
Integrates thoughts, feelings and actions	Displays disharmony between thoughts, feelings and actions
Resolves conflict	Unable to make choices; exercises poor judgement
Relationship With Others	
Establishes and maintains positive relationships	Unable to establish or maintain relationships; uncomfortable with others
Assumes responsibility for terminating those relationships which may be harmful or detrimental	Unable to evaluate or terminate threatening relationships
Validates feelings	Denies and/or projects
Works collaboratively	Is defensive or destructive, isolates self
Accepts compromises	Refuses to compromise, maintains rigidity and resistance
Communicates directly	Secretive, suspicious and distrustful
Uses body gestures to enhance or facilitate communication	Uses body gestures instead of verbal language
Varies content of communication appropriate to the situation	Seldom talks about self or focuses entirely on self and content of communication is limited in scope
Respects others	Disdains others
Relationship With Environment	
Organizes environment	Operates in a disorganized fashion
Exerts control over or modifies immediate environment	Exerts minimum or excessive control; creates a new environment
Adapts to change	Unable to retain objectivity
Engages in planned, thoughtful responsible activity	Behaves impulsively and irresponsibly
Resolves power struggles through cooperation and compromise	Unable to deal with the concept of power and/or authority, resulting in dysfunction and disintegration.

To summarize, the mentally healthy person is an individual who has self-awareness, who likes, respects and accepts himself for what he is, and who acknowledges his limitations and seeks improvement. The reader should be aware that failure to possess one or more of the elements listed under mental health does not connote mental illness. Immaturity or lack of specific elements merely points out areas of inadequacy and decreased potential for optimal functioning.

The following two illustrations are symbolic representations of mental health and mental illness. They depict the outcome of what happens to an individual when he is exposed to either sustained positive nurturing or sustained negative experiences.

implications for nursing

The total spectrum of mental health and mental illness—the identifiable criteria for health and specific symptoms of illness—their significant differences and the vast variations in degrees, the endless possibilities of interpretations of behavior and the deceptive nuances which pervade the communication of thoughts and feelings—serves as a background for the practice of nursing. An awareness of the subtleties involved in human behavior influences the practitioner in the kind of care, the quality of care, and the commitment to caring she provides. The nurse's role involves a dual responsibility of not only the treatment of illness but, equally important, of the prevention of illness.

psychiatric—mental health nursing

Psychiatric-mental health nursing is identified as a specialized field within the practice of nursing. The uniqueness attributed to this specialized field is the priority given to and the emphasis placed on the skillful use of the interpersonal process in the attainment of therapeutic goals. The focus of psychiatric-mental health nursing is both corrective and preventative. It is corrective in that it provides individuals, families or groups who are experiencing various degrees of emotional or psycho-social disequilibrium an opportunity to engage in a therapeutic interactional process. It is preventative in that it endeavors through the educative aspect of the interpersonal process and role model exemplification to preserve equilibrium and promote optimum mental health. Psychiatric-mental health nursing incorporates and reflects the theoretical framework upon which the foundation of all nursing is based.

The practice of psychiatric-mental health nursing requires that the nurse commit herself, without reservation, to the basic concepts implicit within the nursing process, namely, that the patient is a person who has a right to the best possible care and a right to be included in the planning of that care. When we say that the patient is a person, we mean that he is a human being entitled to love, recognition, respect, fulfillment—to all the basic needs which enable the individual to function in his entirety. Nursing care is de-

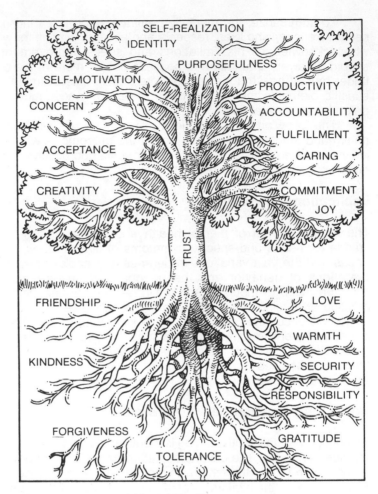

Figure 1-1   *Tree of Mental Health*

signed to utilize these needs in assisting the individual to move toward ac-
tualization of his inherent potential. This concept is the credo by which nurses
must practice. The fundamental satisfaction and gratification the nurse
achieves is based on implementation and realization of this philosophy.

To say that a patient has a right to be included in the planning of his
care is merely extending the idea that the patient is a person, that he has a
right to exert control over his environment and the conditions affecting that
environment in an effort to achieve self-actualization. He is entitled to participate and strive toward the fulfillment of his physical and emotional well-being.
We maintain that a patient is cared for in terms of his totality and not in terms
of his parts. If we believe that patients are human, then we can not talk
around, above, or beneath them, nor can we talk to, for, or about them but
rather, we must talk *with* them.

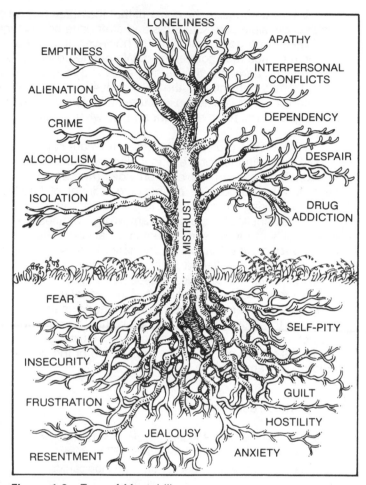

Figure 1-2 *Tree of Mental Illness*

Another concept which we believe is important in developing criteria for care is that behavior has meaning. Here again, we look at the totality of the individual, that is, his spoken words plus the nonverbal ways in which he portrays himself. The two key words of this concept are *behavior* and *meaning*. A broad definition of behavior is that which a person *says and does*. It includes everything! When we use the word *meaning*, we are looking at the implications of the behavior. Meaning may be broadly defined as the way in which an individual attempts to convey the expression of his innermost feeling. We, as nurses, must never lose sight of the fact that what a patient says and does is in response to perceived external and internal stimuli. While the speech and actions of the patient may appear to be without purpose and meaning, they do hold purpose and meaning for the patient. Intervention requires that the nurse be vitally concerned with finding meaning in what is being communicated.

We re-emphasize the concept that the nurse has an obligation to render the best possible care. Students and staff have been taught the rudiments of what makes up good patient care; however, it is the term *obligation* which they sometimes may not perceive. We define obligation as a form of responsibility which demands the nurse's personal investment. It implies the courage of one's convictions, the willingness to give of oneself, the ability to communicate through action and the desire to invest effort into care. The idea of obligation entails the knowledge of what quality care is and how it is provided.

Nursing is a profession involving the care of people. We believe nursing to be a goal-directed process in which the primary objective is to develop a relationship between the care-provider (nurse) and the care-receiver (patient) for the purpose of maintaining a level of health, preventing illness and/or restoring an individual to an optimal level of functioning. Nursing, using a scientific, theoretrical framework, focuses on the uniqueness and individuality of the person. It takes into account the biological, psychosocial and environmental contexts of the patient. Nursing makes use of the interaction between the patient and those with whom he comes in contact. It concerns itself with the significant aspects of the patient's total life experiences. Nursing requires the assessment of individual needs on a personal, interpersonal and intrapersonal level. Nursing modifies the environment to meet the needs of the individual. It produces within the patient a change in attitudes, expectations and possible outcomes. Nursing employs evaluation and judges its effectiveness on the application of the principles derived from the theoretical framework.

suggested readings

Bandman, Bertram and Bandman, Elsie. "Do Nurses Have Rights?" *American Journal of Nursing*, Vol. 78 No. 1 (January, 1978), 84-86.

Cox, Rachel Dunaway. "Concept of Psychological Maturity" in the *American Handbook of Psychiatry*. (2 ed) Aricti Silvano, ed. Vol. I Basic Books: New York, 1974, 214-233.

Goleman, Daniel. "Who's Mentally Ill?" *Psychology Today*, Vol. 11 No. 8 (January, 1978), 34-41.

Jourard, Sidney M. *Healthy Personality: An Approach From The Viewpoint of Humanistic Psychology*. MacMillan Publishing Company, Inc.: New York, 1974.

Katz, Michael. "Making It As A Mental Patient." *Psychology Today*, Vol. 10 (April, 1977), 122-126.

Murray, Ruth and Zentner, Judith. *Nursing Concepts for Health Promotion*. Prentice-Hall, Inc.: Englewood Cliffs, New Jersey, 1975.

Offer, Daniel and Sabskin, Melvin. "Concept of Normality" in the *American Handbook of Psychiatry*. (2 ed) Aricti Silvano, ed. Vol I Basic Books: New York, 202-211.

Price, Joseph L., Drake, Ronald E. and Hine, Lynne Noel. "Value Assumptions in Humanistic Psychiatric Nursing Education." *Perspectives in Psychiatric Care*, Vol. XII No. 2 (1974), 64-69.

Rosenham, D. L. "On Being Sane in Insane Places" in *Psychiatric/Mental Health Nursing: Contemporary Readings*. Backer, Barbara A., Dubbert, Patricia M., Eisenman, Elaine, J. P. D. Van Nostrand Co., Inc.: New York, 1978, 405-426.

Siegel, Hildegarde. "To Your Health—Whatever That May Mean." *Nursing Forum*, Vol. 12 No. 3, 1973, 280-288.

Ventura, Marlene S. "The Dysfunction of D.S.M.-11" in *Psychiatric/Mental Health Nursing: Contemporary Readings*. Backer, Barbara A., Dubbert, Patricia M., Eisenman, Elaine, J. P. D. Van Nostrand Co., Inc.: New York, 1978, 427-433.

Wu, Ruth. *Behavior and Illness*. Prentice-Hall, Inc.: Englewood Cliffs, New Jersey, 1973.

chapter 2

the therapeutic self

learning objectives

On completion of this chapter, the reader should be able to:

1 Develop an understanding of the concept *therapeutic self.*
2 Increase self-awareness through systematic examination of the personal and professional self.
3 Foster growth and development of the therapeutic self.
4 Define the term *attitude* as used throughout this book.
5 Identify those positive attitudes essential in the delivery of nursing care.
6 Demonstrate the use of these attitudes in patient care.
7 Recognize and acknowledge interdisciplinary relationships and their contributions to total patient care as they relate directly and/or indirectly to nursing practice.

The concept of the therapeutic self plays a major role in the development of a positive attitudinal approach to patient care. In this chapter, we will discuss the concept and meaning of the therapeutic self. In addition, we will identify and elaborate on those positive attitudes we feel are a necessary foundation in the nurse's practice and which will promote her appropriate and meaningful intervention with each patient.

the self as a person and as a professional

Reading the phrase *the therapeutic self*, the nurse asks, "What does it mean?" and, "How do I achieve it?" Inherent in this phrase is the idea that I, the nurse, make a difference. Immediately, within the mind there should be an image that I can do something to bring about or effect change. In other words, I am a change agent. What I do, what I say, what I think, and what I feel makes me unique, and my uniqueness is the *key* to caring. If change is to occur, it is up to me to bring it about.

The kind of change I bring about must be positive, that is, I must enable the patient to move toward an optimal health care goal. To achieve this positive change, I must look at myself and examine my assets and liabilities, first as a person, and second, as a professional.

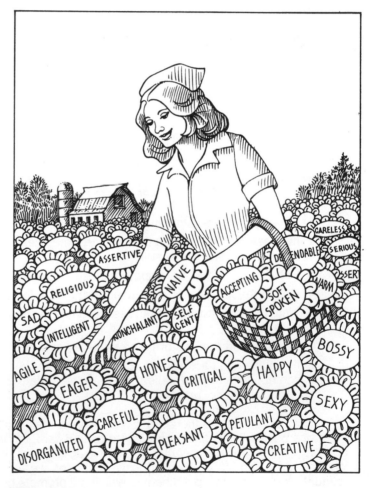

Figure 2-1

First I must examine my characteristics and traits—my total personality. To accomplish this, I must consider the following questions:

What value system do I hold?

What is my level of irritability?

What mood changes do I experience?

Do I have an easygoing attitude toward myself and others?

Do I have a sense of humor?

Am I able to laugh at myself?

What are my habits or patterns relating to my appearance, speech and posture?

What are my reactions to similar or different situations?

Do I underestimate or overestimate my abilities?

Can I made decisions?

Can I accept my shortcomings?

Do I like and respect myself?

How do I relate with others?

How do I see myself in relationship to authority figures, peers, loved ones and strangers?

Am I patient or do I complain excessively?

Am I considerate of others or do I take them for granted?

Do I acknowledge and respect the differences I find in other people?

How do I function within my entire living experience?

Do I exercise my ability to meet my own basic needs in a variety of situations?

Do I deal with problems as they arise?

How open am I to new experiences and new ideas?

Do I make use of my own creative and natural talents?

Am I practical, sensitive, impulsive, idealistic, quiet, reserved, outgoing and/or effervescent?

Your responses to these questions indicate the kind of individual you are and how you function in your daily living. After reviewing these questions, it should become apparent that a qualified practitioner must know herself—her reactions, capabilities and limitations. Armed with this assessment of the personal self, the nurse will be able to proceed to discover the extended and expanded dimensions of the professional self. Without the knowledge gained from an honest appraisal of the personal self, the therapeutic self can be, and is, in jeopardy of being ineffective as a change agent.

Next I must examine the occupational, working segment of my total personality—my professional self. Some questions I must consider:

What is my basic level of knowledge and preparation?

To what extent do I implement my previous learning?

Do I hold myself responsible for my performance?

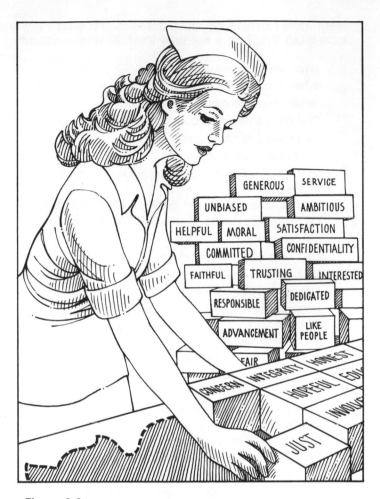

Figure 2-2

What were my reasons for choosing nursing as a career?
What degree of satisfaction do I receive from the work I do?
To what extent do I adhere to my professional code of ethics?
What influences do I exert over the lives of othes and to what degree?
Do I push people around? Do I allow myself to be pushed around?
Can I say no?
Can I set realistic goals for myself and with my patients?
What fears do I have?
What hopes do I express?
What kind of judgments am I called upon to make?
What amount of giving is required of me?
What degree of personal investment must I make and direct toward the
pursuit of increased knowledge?

To complete the examination of the professional self, the nurse also needs to consider the ongoing assessment of daily functioning as a practitioner; the type of relationship established and maintained with nurse colleagues and other professionals; the degree of commitment to the nursing profession; the level of involvement with the professional organization and the level of knowledge about and involvement with the nurse's community and its resources. This personal examination serves as a basis for establishing the nurse's identity and acts as a point of departure for further growth and development of the therapeutic self. In essence, the process outlined above enables the nurse to identify who and what the self is, where the self is, how the self functions and why the self functions as it does.

In addition to the nurse's awareness and knowledge concerning self, there is another dimension to the concept of the therapeutic self. It is the idea of *being yourself*. To be yourself implies recognition of personal strengths and weaknesses and the ability to work with and use them to the best advantage in therapeutic patient care. How does the nurse use an acknowledged strength or weakness constructively? By being genuine, honest, open and flexible. In being herself, the nurse *shares* feelings as opposed to trying to mask or cover them. This sharing is a very meaningful part of honest and open communication. In the process of sharing, the nurse feels free to feel sadness, happiness, loneliness, gladness—free to be as a person. A tear, a hand on the shoulder in comfort, a smile or a joke shared with a patient can convey, as no other means, the reality of the nurse as a person and as a professional. This humanness is the essence of professionalism.

However, being yourself does not give the nurse license to forget, deny or abuse basic principles, or to act impulsively without thought for the consequences, or to relate *every* personal experience with the patient. Being yourself means being your professional self, that is, bringing to the therapeutic situation all the knowledge, skill and judgment that can assist, support and encourage the patient to move toward health. The therapeutic self is that personal awareness, knowledge, and understanding which when put into operation results in a positive experience for the patient, his family, and his community.

specific positive attitudes

The operational or internalized concept of the therapeutic self permits the nurse to develop those positive attitudes which will enable her to provide the best possible nursing care. In many nursing texts where the student is instructed to develop positive attitudes for patient care, we find such terms as *friendliness, matter-of-factness, permissiveness* and *reassurance.* These terms are the type of approach the nurse is to use; that is, they are what the nurse does as opposed to the attitudes the nurse holds. By *attitude* we mean the opinion or view the nurse has toward patients, hospitalization, caring, colleagues, life and death. Some of the necessary attitudes the nurse must cultivate in approaching patients are the attitudes of personal worth, integrity, open-mindedness, advocacy, hopefulness and involvement.

An attitude of *personal worth* is the viewpoint the nurse holds about self and others. The basis for this attitude is the extent of the nurse's awareness and understanding of such things as cultural differences and social influences affecting people, respect for humanity and tolerance and patience toward human frailty. For example, the nurse displays an attitude of personal worth when she anticipates and acknowledges religious eating habits and adapts hospital service to meet the needs of the individual, when she provides privacy and comfort for a patient undergoing a physical examination or when she explains completely to the patient, more than once if necessary, any procedures he must undergo. The nurse's approach should demonstrate a conviction that the dignity, individuality and equality of people must be protected at all costs. With this kind of framework, then, the nurse does not approach a patient in a rigid, stereotyped fashion.

When we say that the nurse must demonstrate an attitude of *personal integrity,* we mean that the nurse maintains an honesty toward herself in her dealings with herself and with others. An old but still viable cliché which conveys our meaning quite clearly is: "To thine own self be true." Demonstration of this attitude makes visible the code of ethics under which the nurse operates and which in all conscience cannot be violated. Integrity of the self implies that the nurse is just, fair, honest, dependable and conscientious and willing and able to acknowledge commitment to the profession, to patients and to self. Personal integrity demands that the nurse accepts challenge, responsibility, accountability and is committed to a willingness to take risks.

Open-mindedness is an attitude which conveys the idea that a willingness to change is present within the nurse. She is ready to adapt and be flexible. Open-mindedness is an attitude which permits the nurse to really hear what is being said despite the fact that she may hold a contrary opinion. Open-mindedness is accepting the right of others to hold values and make decisions which may differ from one's own. To develop an attitude of open-mindedness the nurse should continuously ask herself *why, how, what* and *under what circumstances*?

Advocacy as an attitude for the nurse is a relatively new and challenging idea. Advocacy is an attitude of support which safeguards the rights and integrity of the patient. It demands that the nurse expand the health concept of doing unto a person for his own good to include *standing up* for the good of the patient. When a nurse takes the attitude of advocacy, she supports the patient in those decisions he feels are right and necessary for the maintenance of his personal integrity. Advocacy is a matter of fighting for the good of the patient; it is never undertaken when the outcome may be harmful to the patient's total welfare. When the situation may be harmful either physically or emotionally, such as when a patient who has made a suicidal gesture wants to leave the hospital or terminate therapy against professional judgment, the nurse cannot advocate such a decision. In such a situation advocacy would require that the nurse seek support from nurse colleagues as well as professionals from other disciplines to sustain therapeutic intervention.

Mrs. Small, a 43-year old divorced, Caucasian female, was admitted to the psychiatric unit of a hospital following a six-month period of increasing depression and inability to function adequately as a legal secretary and as a mother of two teen-age children. She refused to go to work, prepare meals or do household chores. She spent her days in bed and complained of crying for no apparent reason. After three weeks of this behavior, her family physician suggested that Mrs. Small seek psychiatric consultation. As a result, she was hospitalized for psychiatric treatment.

After eight days of hospitalization, Mrs. Small stated that she was "feeling better" and had received "much needed rest." She thought she was ready to return to her job and her children, who were being cared for by her mother. Mrs. Pryor, a staff nurse, encouraged Mrs. Small to remain in the hospital for further treatment and therapeutic intervention that might then be followed through an out-patient basis. Mrs. Small insisted on being discharged and was verbally abusive of other patients and the psychiatrist. She repeatedly declared herself "not crazy," became agitated and frequently burst into tears.

Mrs. Pryor had observed and charted Mrs. Small's loss of sleep, restlessness during the day, poor appetite and consequent weight loss. Mrs. Small remained in bed most of the day and refused to participate in any therapeutic or recreational activities on the ward. Nonetheless, Mrs. Small insisted on her discharge and demanded release as "her right" since she had been hospitalized voluntarily. Mrs. Pryor increased her contacts with Mrs. Small and allowed the patient to ventilate and share her feelings. At the same time Mrs. Pryor informed and consulted with the psychiatrist, the psychologist, the clinical social worker and the other nurses about these developments. Mrs. Pryor felt that Mrs. Small was still depressed and was possibly a suicidal risk so that she could not advocate and support Mrs. Small's request for a discharge from the hospital. Mrs. Pryor shared with the treatment team that she respected the right of the patient to make decisions but was concerned for Mrs. Small's physical and emotional well-being if she were to leave the hospital. The treatment team agreed with Mrs. Pryor and together they formulated a plan of intervention to assist Mrs. Small to work through her crisis. The psychiatrist re-evaluated Mrs. Small's medication and intensified his supervision of psychotropic intervention; the psychologist agreed to contact the legal firm which employed Mrs. Small in order to assess her functioning on the job and to plan for whatever testing that might be necessary for her vocational rehabilitation. The clinical social worker agreed to contact Mrs. Small's mother and request support for continued hospitalization and reassurance about the children's well-being. The family was encouraged to visit. Mrs. Pryor was to assume the role as primary therapist with Mrs. Small and would see her on a daily basis.

Mrs. Small reluctantly agreed to remain in the hospital for a maximum of three more weeks. During one of the therapy sessions with Mrs. Pryor, Mrs. Small admitted that she was feeling anxious, overwhelmed and discouraged since she felt she was not improving rapidly enough and was, in fact, contemplating going home to commit suicide.

During the next three weeks Mrs. Small showed a marked improvement in her affect, appearance, appetite and sleep pattern. She began to converse with the staff and other patients and she participated in group discussions and recreational activities. She stated she enjoyed the visits from her parents and children and had telephoned her employers to discuss her future with them. Mrs. Small was subsequently discharged from the hospital. Mrs. Pryor arranged for her to continue therapy on an out-patient basis at the Neighborhood mental health clinic. Mrs. Small returned to her job and with assistance enrolled in art school two evenings a week.

This actual case history serves an an example of effective advocacy and demonstrates the intervention of the nurse on behalf of the patient. Note that Mrs. Pryor acknowledges the patient's insistence on discharge and her ability to maintain objectivity in view of the patient's demands, negativism and verbal abuse.

To further illustrate the attitude of advocacy, let us look at a situation in which the nurse is caring for a patient who has difficulty in his home situation in addition to the medical problems for which he is seeking care. The nurse has identified aspects of the problem which lie beyond the realm of a nurse's capabilities and expertise. The nursing action at this point would require a recommendation to the patient that a social agency could be of assistance. Previously, nurses have been told that they stop there and leave the rest up to the patient. However, a patient advocate would provide him with a list of names and telephone numbers and might even phone for him. What if the nurse finds that after making the recommendation, the patient vehemently opposes the recommendation? The nurse's attitude of advocacy demands supporting him in his decision to reject the services of the agency and, at the same time, exploring with the patient possible alternatives which might be more acceptable.

Another attitude that is essential for the nurse to cultivate in approaching patients is that of *hopefulness.* Hopefulness is looking at a situation from the bright side. By no means do we propose a Pollyanna attitude. What we do advocate is that the nurse feel within herself an optimism, a recognition that professional attitudes, knowledge and skills do make a difference, that even in the most hopeless of situations, the nurse can use this knowledge and skill to be of support and bring peace and comfort to the patient and assist the patient to find meaning in his illness. Hopefulness is conveyed through touch, "bright shining eyes," a "light step," a warm smile and a kind, interested word. These and other such actions on the part of the nurse convey to the patient that here is a human being who knows what life and death is all about and whose care and attention demonstrates concern. The message of hope is subtly transmitted through commitment to caring.

The last of the attitudes we would like to call attention to is that of *involvement.* Involvement demands a personal and professional responsibility of the highest order. The attitude of involvement means that the nurse places priority first on the practice of nursing and last on the self. This does not mean that the nurse is not concerned about her economic welfare, working conditions and other personal conditions which may affect the nurse's total well-being. It does mean that in the day-to-day operation of professional activities, the nurse functions to the best of her ability regardless of the personal circumstances in which she finds herself. It also means that if the circumstances are such that they may result in poor practice, lack of safety for the patient or disregard for professional ethics, the nurse is obliged to use whatever means available to rectify the circumstances.

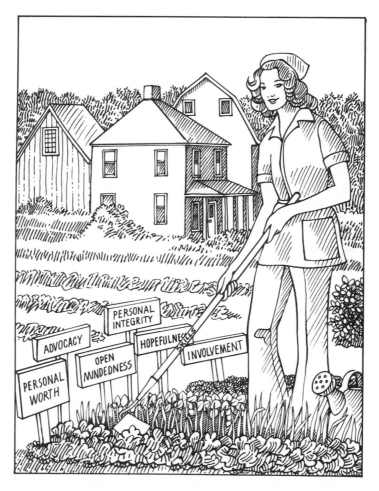

Figure 2-3

In this chapter we have presented our concept of the therapeutic self and the attitudes essential for development of a mental health approach to patient care. It is our firm belief that these concepts are the most viable tools needed by a nurse in any fundamental area of practice or level of patient care responsibility. It is up to the nurse to recognize and cultivate the unique, individual, personal and professional potentialities of self.

suggested readings

Bindschadler, Helga Proctel. "Dare To Be You." American Journal of Nursing Vol. 76, No. 10 (October, 1976), 1632-1633.

Brill, Naomi I. *Working With People: The Helping Process.* J. B. Lippincott Company: Philadelphia, 1978.

Fay, Patricia. "Sounding Board: In Support of Patient Advocacy As A Nursing Role." *Nursing Outlook* Vol. 26 No. 4 (April, 1978), 252-253.

Folta, Jeannette, and Duke, Edith, eds. *A Sociological Framework for Patient Care.* John Wiley & Sons Inc.: New York, 1966.

Frankl, Viktor E. *Man's Search for Meaning.* Washington Square Press: New York, 1969.

King, Edwina Skiba, R. N. "Should We Get Emotionally Involved? Hell Yes!" *R.N. Magazine* Vol. 40 (June, 1977), 48-53.

Kramer, Marlene, and Schmalenberg, Claudia. *Path To Biculturalism.* Contemporary Publishing, Inc.: Wakefield, Massachusetts, 1977.

LaMonica, Elaine L., et al. "Empathy Training as the Major Thrust of a Staff Development Program." *Nursing Research* Vol. 25 No. 6 (November-December 1976), 447-451.

Maloney, Elizabeth. *Interpersonal Relations.* Wm. C. Brown: Dubuque, Iowa, 1966.

Mlott, Sylvester R. "Personality Correlates of a Psychiatric Nurse." *Journal of Psychiatric and Mental Health Services* Vol. 14 No. 2 (February, 1976), 19-23.

Neylan, Margaret Prowse. "The Nurse in a Helping Milieu." *American Journal of Nursing* Vol. 61 No. 4 (April, 1961), 72-74.

Peplau, Hildegard E. "An Open Letter to a New Graduate." *Nursing Digest* (March-April 1975), 36-37.

Quinn, Nancy, and Somers, Anne R. "The Patient's Bill of Rights." *Nursing Outlook,* Vol. 22 No. 4 (April, 1974), 240-244.

Rogers, Carl R. *On Becoming A Person.* Houghton Mifflin Company: Boston, 1961, 19-23.

Shikora-Wachter, Nancy. "Scapegoating Among Professionals." *American Journal of Nursing,* Vol. 77 No. 3 (March, 1977), 406-409.

Sinkier, Gail H. "Identity and Role." *Nursing Outlook,* Vol. 18 No. 10 (October, 1970), 22-24.

Smith, Lovetta L. " 'to be, or not to be . . .' " *Journal of Psychiatric Nursing and Mental Health Services XV,* No. 10 (October, 1977), 37-39.

Smoyak, Shirley A. "The Confrontation Process." *American Journal of Nursing,* Vol. 74, No. 9 (September 1974), 1632-1635.

chapter 3

communication: method—process—practice

learning objectives

On completion of this chapter the reader should be able to:

1 Define the term *communication*.
2 Distinguish between *social* and *therapeutic communication*.
3 Identify and describe the operational definition of the communication process.
4 Identify the barriers to effective communication.
5 List the three major categories into which effective communication practices may be divided.
6 Identify the specific nursing behavior associated with each of the communication categories.
7 Understand how the therapeutic techniques of communication are used.

The concepts and practices of communication play a significant role in the social interactional process among people. As a therapeutic tool, communication becomes an even more significant adjunct within the therapeutic interactional process. In this chapter, we will synthesize and clarify those aspects which are fundamental to the nurse's understanding of just what communication is and, most importantly, of how both the nurse and the patient can benefit from its successful application.

We present this material with the hope that the nurse can come to a better understanding of the importance communication plays in the development of the therapeutic self.

definition of communication

Communication is a frequently used term in today's society. Everybody's "communicating" but just what are they doing? What exactly is communication? We know that communication is a *process*, a logical, step-by-step progression of operations directed toward specific expected outcomes. As such, communication is the means we use to relate and share our thoughts, feelings, attitudes, needs, desires, pains, turmoils and crises to others. The process of communication uses words and expressions which can be interpreted or heard differently. Communication takes place between people and can be either verbal or nonverbal.

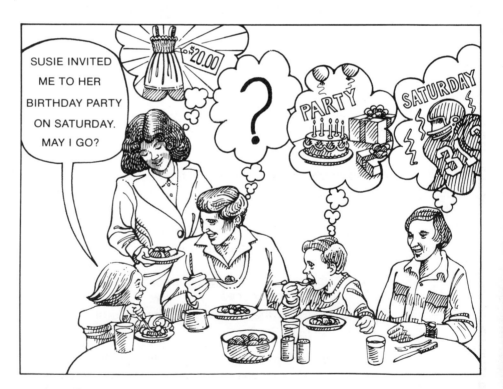

Figure 3-1

We know that communication is instrumental in achieving satisfaction and aids in the solution of problems. We also know that communication can be a source of distress or discomfort. But, what else is it?

Communication is:

A dynamic social process involving an exchange of ideas between two or more people.

A behavior used to express feelings.

A system of operations that includes language, gestures, or symbols to convey intended meaning.

A method by which information is transmitted, received and understood.

A mutual transactional process used to facilitate a relationship with others.

An essential element in the establishment of the nurse-patient relaionship.

therapeutic communication

Therapeutic communication differs from the usual social communicative process in that in therapeutic communication the messages which are sent and received are designed to deal with presenting problems and dissatisfactions from stressful living situations, learning to use or increase coping abilities, and developing and fortifying ego strengths. The thrust of this form of communication is to create a space for the patient to engage in learning experiences—a physical and emotional space free of the encumbrances which result from the pressure of "aloneness and helplessness" the patient often feels when confronting a problem or crisis. The nurse initiates a focusing on the identified needs and goals of the patient. These are given priority throughout the therapeutic process and, because of its dynamic nature, the process requires continuous re-evaluation which can result in revision of priorities or goals and in assisting the patient to reorder his needs and desires. Another unique characteristic of the therapeutic communication process is that as the process continues and evolves the patient assumes a more active verbal and/or nonverbal communicative role.

principles for effective communication

We have identified at least four basic criteria the nurse can use to determine whether or not effective communication is achieved between herself and her patient.

First, the nurse recognizes that verbal and body language mean different things to different people. Too many times, people take for granted that the words they choose to use to express themselves are understood exactly as intended. This is not so. It is well-known that a majority of problems people encounter center on misunderstanding and misinterpretation of communications. For communication to be clear and direct, the words must be mutually understood to sender and receiver. Therefore, it is important for the nurse to choose those words which have the most universal understanding and application. The nurse must consider and ask herself, does this word or phrase apply to this particular situation, and have meaning for this person? Could misunderstanding be avoided by a more careful selection of terms? For example, if someone said to us, "Look out," our immediate response would be to look for an environmental threat. We would most likely not go to the window and "look out."

The nurse must periodically check with the patient to determine if the messages are received and are understood. The nurse can do this simply by asking him if he understands or the nurse can request that the patient tell her, in his own words, the essence of the message. The nurse must also observe for nonverbal responses such as a change in the tone of voice which might be indicative of misunderstanding. The nurse's responsibility then takes the form of encouraging the patient to express his concern, voice his doubts and question what he does not understand.

Second, the nurse recognizes the presence of patterns in the transmission and reception of messages. Just as words have specific meanings, so too does the way in which these words are put together in transmission and in reception have meaning. Identification of patterns is essential if communication between the nurse and her patient is to be clear and explicit.

An individual learns through the developmental process a particular mode of expression. He communicates discomfort, distress, anxiety, hostility and other feelings through a particular communication pattern he has set up with others. Reliance on this pattern becomes habitual. Such patterns of behavior often interfere with the open-minded sending and receiving of messages. Therefore, the nurse should know to observe for such patterns as the kind and amount of emphasis placed on particular words; the repetitive use of words or phrases; changes in tonal quality and pitch when specific subjects are discussed; or body movements indicating an approach toward or retreat from the sender.

If the nurse identifies the presence of patterns both within herself and within the patient, she is in a better position to achieve the specific purpose of the communication. For example, an individual who consciously or unconsciously wishes to avoid revealing information about self, will either tend to place himself in a side-to-side communication position as opposed to selecting a face-to-face seating arrangement or he will not engage in direct eye contact with the nurse. The nurse's awareness and recognition of this pattern of behavior allows her an opportunity to validate the impressions received. It also provides the nurse with an opportunity to focus on an area that might have a great deal of significant meaning for the patient.

Third, the nurse recognizes the importance personal experiences play in the interpretation of communication. An individual's perception of what is communicated is colored by his present and past experiences as well as his future expectations. For example, after the death of a family member a period of grieving occurs in which the surviving member(s) feels a sense of loss and sadness. However, suppose the deceased family member was a domineering, self-centered, caustic, intimidating and manipulative individual. In this situation, the survivor(s) may not view the death as a loss, but may instead experience a sense of freedom and relief. If so, it would be erroneous for the nurse to assume that the survivor is mourning and "putting up a good front." In other words, the nurse cannot assume that generalities apply to a particular set of circumstances. The nurse must know the patient as a person and understand him within his own frame of reference before valid interpretations can be made.

Fourth, the nurse recognizes the degree to which her patient can abstract and conceptualize as part of the communication process. The ability to abstract and conceptualize demands a high level of intellectual functioning. Individuals are endowed with variations of this ability. Environmental situations, psychological causes and/or physiological changes are also responsible for variations. Effective communication requires that the individual internalize the message. The resultant appropriate response to the message demonstrates this internalization through discrimination and exercise of judgment in filtering out the pertinent from the unpertinent.

The nurse who engages in a therapeutic relationship must be aware of the possible levels of abstraction and conceptualization so that she can set realistic expectations. Often the patient can only think concretely; that is, his ability to abstract is almost non existent. This is true of patients diagnosed as being mentally retarded, having an organic brain syndrome, or having sustained early culturosocial, emotional deprivation. In psychotic patients we often find that internalization of transactions related to the environment is extreme and, consequently, they lose contact with or avoid reality and often develop a delusional or hallucinatory system to deliberately minimize their multisensory input.

It is appropriate for the nurse to initiate goals that are limited in scope and that can be achieved by the individual. Adequate recognition on the part of the nurse prevents communication from becoming a frustrating process as opposed to a therapeutic process. In the mental health field one of the most frequent errors of psychotherapeutic intervention is that many professionals tend to analyze every word, action or body movement. This technique may be detrimental to the patient because it can lead to the professional misinterpreting the messages communicated or losing the objective ability to understand and work through relevant data with the patient. It is of vital importance to the successful outcome of the therapeutic communicative engagement that the nurse learn to see and assess what messages are significant, to what degree, and what to accept at face value.

To evaluate the effectiveness of communication, the nurse must consciously and thoughtfully apply each of the above principles. If any one of the principles is omitted in the assessment process, the nurse is left with an incomplete picture of the patient's understanding of what is being communicated. This incomplete picture may incorrectly and negatively influence the nurse's interpretation of the patient's needs. It may also produce barriers to communication which may tend to decrease or retard the establishment of trust and rapport. This decrease could result in prolonging the patient's need for therapy.

the communication process—operational definition

Communication is a complex art that requires learning and mastery. Therapeutic communication is based on the application of a set of principles. The principles are used as guidelines in the development of the structure and form involved in the communicative process. The process itself depends on the application of therapeutic techniques which are used to facilitate the movement of the participants toward the identified goal. No one is born with the knowledge and ability to be therapeutic. Acquisition of principles and skills is not automatic. Therapeutic communication is hard work and demands that the nurse be actively involved. How? By requiring that the nurse demonstrate sensitivity toward others and a willingness to give of self. This sensitivity and willingness to share self occurs as the nurse comes to an awareness of who she is as a person, where she is at any moment, how she arrived there, the set of values she holds, the knowledge of what she is able to achieve and the degree to which she can extend herself.

The communication process is composed of a series of six operations in which the nurse assumes an active, dynamic role. Meaningful communication cannot occur unless these operations are put into practice in each nurse-patient interaction. They are described below.

1) be there

To be there the nurse must be fully conscious and aware of the purpose of the interaction. It requires that the nurse's full attention is focused on the individual(s) with whom she is interacting. Accessibility and availability do not fulfill the requirements of "being there." *"Being there"* implies interest, expectancy, readiness and attentiveness. These qualities can be demonstrated by such nursing behaviors as ignoring and/or eliminating distractions, looking directly at the patient as opposed to gazing about the room, remaining quietly composed as opposed to fidgeting in the chair, sitting erect and slightly forward as opposed to leaning back and away from the patient, and giving verbal encouragement for the patient to begin the interaction.

2) observe

Standing about, looking around and sitting in a nurse's station are patterns of behavior engaged in by many nurses under the guise of observation; however, this is not therapeutic observation. *Observation* is deliberate, planned and systematized. To observe is to see the total patient. It is a data-gathering process that requires accuracy and objectivity in seeing the individual as a person who is separate and distinct from others as he functions within the context of his reality and environment.

Observation is the process of obtaining objective and subjective data. In objective data gathering the nurse makes use of her multisensory inputs— information gained through the five basic senses together with the information gained through specific nursing techniques or procedures, such as taking the patient's vital signs in an attempt to assess the patient's physical and emotional functioning. In subjective data gathering the nurse employs the therapeutic communicative techniques to elicit from the patient his perceptions of himself and his functioning. Within the context of the nurse-patient interaction, to observe is to be cognizant of responses and to look for cues and patterns with regard to the patient's feelings, thoughts and behavior.

3) listen

Listening is the art of paying attention to the speaker. Many nurses hear and do not listen, that is, they hear only what they want to hear. To listen demands a great deal of effort and concentration. It also requires sensitivity to words, tonal qualities, silences, hidden messages with significant content, generalizations and unrecognized feelings. To listen the nurse must actively seek to reduce environmental and personal distractions.

Listening, like observation, requires objectivity and accuracy. There are four major types of listening processes: defensive, selective, deliberative and empathic. The nurse's understanding of each of these forms of listening is important because it helps her develop better use of the therapeutic self, aids and ameliorates the communicative process and facilitates the establishment of rapport with the patient.

Defensive listening is the process of hearing by either filtering the messages so as to hear only that which is perceived or to place personal and negative values on the message. This type of listening inhibits spontaneity and rapport. A patient often is prepared "to hear the worst" or to be "accused" by the nurse, resulting in misinterpretation or confusion. The sources of defensive listening are often guilt, shame, fear and feelings of inadequacy or worthlessness. The sources of this type of listening are the same for all, nurse or patient. When a nurse engages in defensive listening she prevents the real message from being heard and distorts its meaning. We devoted Chapter 2 to the development of the therapeutic self because an honest assessment of the self greatly minimizes defensive listening and allows the nurse to understand and explore defensive listening with the patient.

Selective listening is an inherent practice. We all like to hear what we want to hear, even though it may not have been said by the other person. Also, we have the habit of hearing only part of what is being said or communicated. Figure 3-1 is a good example of what occurs in selective listening. In this illustration the young girl delivered an explicit message and asked a clear question. Members of the family heard what they wanted to hear and the father heard nothing at all. What family members perceived to hear is what is called selective listening. Hence, it is obvious that arbitrary selective listening in the therapeutic setting is detrimental.

Deliberate listening may accompany selective listening. Often one hears the expression, "I heard every word he said!" to emphasize that the listener got the message clearly, distinctly and without error. Another example is that of the listener replying, "I understand." Both of these statements illustrate the deliberate attentiveness of the listener and demonstrate the absence of defensive and selective hearing. They represent a type of hearing that excludes placing personal value judgments upon what is being said. *Attentiveness* is the essence of deliberate listening. In therapy deliberate listening is vital. If the patient knows he is being heard and understood he is at ease, his anxiety decreases and he willingly volunteers more information about himself and his emotions. On the other hand, the patient must also learn deliberate listening. To assist in developing this type of listening the nurse must, especially when discussing very significant data, be sure to validate that the patient has understood. If not, the question or statement should be clarified until the message is received and understood.

Empathic listening is the core of therapeutic intervention. To state it simply, it means to listen with empathy. It includes the ability to feel and understand what the patient is saying without losing objectivity. Empathic listening also means to just listen to what the person has to say and proffer no comments unless directly requested to do so. Further clarification of empathy may be found in Chapter Five.

4) respond

It is not uncommon to find a nurse responding to a patient with hackneyed phrases. This occurs because of "non-thereness," inadequate observation and inattentive listening. The resultant communication is ineffective, inaccurate and misrepresentative. *To respond* is to indicate to the sender, either verbally or nonverbally, that the message is received but is not necessarily understood. It is an opportunity to talk and to share. A response may take many forms and serve many purposes. It may be used to supply information in answer to a question; express mutual understanding derived from an empathetic experience; provide a greeting in acknowledgment or recognition; ask for clarification of issues and viewpoints; or provide feedback in the promotion of understanding. In responding, the nurse assumes the responsibility of helping the patient clarify the meaning and intent of his verbal and non verbal expressions. The response of the nurse is not an impulsive reaction. It is the thoughtful and selective application of knowledge to the particular situation at a given moment. If the response is acceptable, the communication process continues uninterrupted and leads to goal fulfillment. If the response is unacceptable, communication may break down.

5) interpret

The nurse can alienate and isolate a patient by making a too-rapid interpretation. *To interpret* is to derive meaning from that which is being communicated. The interpretation process is accomplished through a mutual sharing and exploration of data. Accurate and valid interpretation requires time, effort and patience. The explicit and implicit meanings that are conveyed to the sender are not always clear; therefore, interpretation depends on the nurse's application of her knowledge of individual lifestyles as well as her understanding and acceptance of differences. The degree to which the nurse is able to consider various possible interpretations depends to a large extent on her ability to feel comfortable with her own words and with the language or modes of expression used by the patient. Interpretation requires that the nurse display honesty and sincerity in the search for meaning, since any artificiality in the nurse's approach is almost always immediately detected and viewed as a negative response by the patient. Inaccurate interpretation is a disservice to the patient because it may contribute to the acceptance of erroneous information as fact or may cause the patient to set up resistance to the interaction process.

6) validate

The last and most complex operation in the communication process is validation. Once the nurse selects the most significant of all possible interpretations of the communicated message, she is in a position to present these to the patient for verification. *To validate* is to corroborate or substantiate the interpretations that have been made within the context of the nurse-patient interaction. It is an ongoing process. In most situations, interpretations need immediate validation, as in the case of feelings which may be implied but not directly expressed, or when the nurse suspects a different usage for a particular word or phrase. In other instances, presentation of interpretations to the patient for validation depends on the readiness of the patient to accept and use the validated material in a constructive manner. Because readiness is a critical factor affecting change and goal achievement, timing is of utmost importance in the execution of the validation process.

Not only does the nurse validate her interpretations with the patient, she also seeks to validate them with colleagues and/or supervisors. The purpose of this aspect of validation is twofold. First, it enables the nurse to maintain her objectivity. Second, it provides a means by which the nurse can follow through on the critical analyses and evaluation of the interaction process in light of her performance and in view of the stated therapeutic goals. It is through the active pursuit for validation that the nurse can realistically assess and perfect her skills in communication, thereby permitting her to grow, experience personal and professional satisfaction and increase her therapeutic effectiveness.

The communication process is a step-by-step dynamic procedure used in both social and therapeutic communication. The responsibility for initiating and maintaining therapeutic communication rests with the nurse. With her also remains the obligation to follow each step of the process, regardless of the patient's initial ability to participate. In the application of the process the nurse must exercise judgment and move only as the patient is able to move. If the communication process is followed and practiced in normal day-to-day living, there would be little need for the establishment of therapeutic communication.

communication barriers

As human beings we never cease to communicate; however, that which we communicate is not always clearly understood. A variety of internal and external factors influence the manner in which the message is sent, received and comprehended. If the communicator is unaware of these factors and their influence on the communicative process, he is unable to deal with them. The net result is a breakdown in the communication process. For clarity and understanding, we identify four major barriers to communication. Encompassed in these are a majority of the most common internal and external factors influencing communication.

1) inaccurate perception of self and/or others

As with every other facet of living, knowledge of self is a prerequisite for communication. A person's attitudes, beliefs and values shape the transmission, reception and understanding of conscious and unconscious messages. A breakdown occurs when an individual assumes that his attitudes, beliefs and values are shared by another. And even if there are similarities, because of individual differences, they will not be identical. Variations should be expected and given consideration. For example, two middle-class mothers, Mother A and Mother B, each with a family of four, verablize to each other about the necessity to practice economy in a world of rising costs. Both talk of clipping coupons and taking advantage of "good buys." From their conversation, you would initially gather that both women shop in the same manner. In talking further with Mother A, you find that she shops at one store and points out savings in terms of gasoline, time and energy. While in talking with Mother B, you find that she does her weekly shopping at several stores and points out savings in terms of a wider selection, redemption stamps and self-satisfaction about "getting bargains." Economy is a shared value and both women take for granted that the other shops in the same way. However, the manner in which they practice economy and the beliefs they hold regarding attainment are markedly different. A question that might well be asked at this point is: Why didn't they go into more detail with each other? The answer is that because each valued economy and shared similar practices they "assumed" that the other carried out all shopping habits in a like manner and thereby didn't explore further.

Another example to illustrate what happens when there is inaccurate perception of self and others in the therapeutic situation is one which involves misinterpretation of role.

As part of the student's clinical experience in a psychiatric setting a nursing student has been assigned to a patient, Mr. X. The patient has been informed that a nursing student will be talking with him. When the student approached Mr. S, she introduced herself and stated the reason for her daily contacts with him. Mr. X indicated that he understood and they proceeded to discuss his reasons for being hospitalized. Subsequently, the student accompanied Mr. X to his activities in order to complete the observation and assessment of his functioning. Mr. X began to shift his perception of the student from the professional role to one of a "friendly visitor." His perception became even further distorted as he viewed the student nurse as a "girl friend." The student became upset and consulted her instructor.

This distortion occurred because the nursing student failed to establish and repeatedly clarify her role with Mr. X in this learning experience. Thus, she placed herself and the therapeutic alliance in jeopardy by assuming that Mr. X would continue to remember her role after being provided with only one explanation.

Little or no understanding of one's own attitudes, values and beliefs produces communication breakdown through the expression of inconsistencies. These inconsistencies in words and behavior lead to sending mixed messages which, in turn, result in confusion and misunderstanding by the receiver. They also detract from the credibility of the sender. We use clichés to describe an individual who demonstrates this type of communication breakdown: "She talks out of both sides of her mouth"; "You never know where you stand with her—you're damned if you do, and damned if you don't"; or "Actions speak louder than words." These inconsistencies may also be responsible for engendering within the receiver feelings of irritation, impatience, anger and perhaps even disgust or distrust. Communication cannot survive where such negative feelings exist.

Lack of self-knowledge or knowledge of another with regard to attitudes, beliefs or values provides a medium for the development of bias and prejudice. The natural response displayed by an individual confronted with the possible existence of a bias or prejudice is to deny its presence. Refusal to acknowledge the possibility of bias or prejudice defeats communication in that it produces a closed circuit. The individual is unable either to send or receive accurate messages surrounding a particular person, situation or set of circumstances.

Inaccurate perception of self or another may be produced by other internal and external factors such as one's concern for status and prestige. Status and prestige are equated by some with power—power of position, expertise, competence or force. Breakdown in communication occurs as a result of the misinterpretation or misuse of power. Take for example, the individual who is preoccupied with creating an impression of importance, superior knowledge, competence or wealth. This individual may dwell on his social standing, educational background, credentials or success in the stock market. This type of communication, because of excessive egocentricity turns people off, and thereby negates any avenue for positive communication.

Due to ethnic and cultural background, an individual has a built-in value system. Yet he may not clearly understand that he operates under the imposed traditions and values of that system. Those with whom the individual attempts to communicate also operate under the influence of an inherent ethnic and cultural social system. Operation without recognition of and consideration for self or another leads to the formation of barriers in communication. Such things as the specific language used by a group may not be clearly understood or may be understood in a different context than intended. Pronunciation, accent or word connotations may interfere with the communication process.

The two illustrations that follow graphically portray the difficulties associated with linguistics and the nurse's need to be alert to such potential situations.

> Mrs. Ruiz, a native of Puerto Rico, was admitted to the hospital for observation following complaints of severe abdominal pain. A nursing student was assigned to assist with Mrs. Ruiz's admission to the medical floor of a large metropolitan hospital. The student delivered the prepackaged bedside equipment; as she put each item in place she named each for Mrs. Ruiz—bath basin, kidney basin, water pitcher, soap dish, etc. Later, when the student returned to the room, she found Mrs. Ruiz trying to void in the kidney basin. Upon questioning, Mrs. Ruiz stated that since she had been told it was a kidney basin she used it to relieve her kidneys.

Many times communication is closed down because the sounds are "funny," or confused with other words. Here is an actual incident:

> Tommy, age 5, was being oriented to the pediatric unit following his admission for a tonsillectomy. During the process of acquainting him with his new environment the nurse pointed out several areas, including the linen chute. Tommy's eyes got very big and he turned to look at her in amazement. As they proceeded to walk Tommy reached toward the nurse and tugged at her uniform. When the nurse looked at him he asked, "How do you shoot linen in there?"

2) failure to focus on message or sender

Barriers to communication found in this category result from the listener's inability to zero in on the concerns and messages the sender wishes to convey. Sometimes, in an effort to establish a commonality in the communication bond, speakers frequently change topics to an extent that neither party is able to derive meaning from the messages. The outcome is a sender and receiver who both experience an increased level of frustration and who move away from, instead of toward establishing rapport.

Feelings of inadequacy, real or imagined, prevent an individual from achieving desired communication. This inability produces within the individual anger or hostility which he directs toward the self or projects onto another. Various kinds of "cut-off" behaviors result from these feelings.

One type of "cut-off" behavior is the expression of impatience. Impatient behavior is evidenced by continuous verbal interruptions—when the listener says he understands or already knows, even before the speaker is finished talking, or by such nonverbal behavior as turning away from the communicator, responding to distractions in the environment or using facial expressions which convey boredom or disinterest in the message. Through these behaviors, the receiver is telling the sender to "hurry along and get it over with." When this happens there is a failure to pick up on the key words or cues which are indicative of the sender's main concern. Further progression toward goal attainment is then blocked.

Prying is another manifestation of "cut-off" behavior. Prying is an attempt to uncover material irrelevant to the sender's main message, which he is not ready to reveal. It may be asking for details—gory or sexual—that have no relation to the problem or process but merely gratify the curiosity of the receiver. Prying is destructive and dehumanizing because the individual seeking therapeutic intervention is made to feel that he cannot retain the right to withold non-pertinent information. It demonstrates disrespect, disinterest and unconcern for the individual. A patient is sensitive to this unprofessional behavior and frequently expresses negative feelings about the receiver to others. The only purpose that prying serves is to satisfy one's need for power, control and/or gratification of one's own needs. Often the information gleaned from prying is used by the nurse as subject material for gossip among other professionals.

Failure to focus on the sender or the message is the outcome of inattentive listening. It is another form of communication block. Inattentive listening is selective hearing, that is, hearing what one wants to hear when it is convenient to hear it. Inattentive listening is one of the most prevalent pitfalls occurring in ordinary, everyday communication. Just consider the following excerpt of a conversation between husband and wife. When the wife reminds her husband that the basement needs to be cleaned on Saturday, he acknowledges the message with a nod of his head, apparently indicating that he heard what was said. On Saturday, as he prepares to leave for a golf game with his buddies, his wife asks him about the cleaning project. His response to her is "Why didn't you remind me sooner?" The wife replies, "But I did! On Thursday!" Sound familiar? Or, how about children who are engrossed in a television program before supper and have not heard Mother say, "It's time to set the table!" But, if she had said instead, "There's a bag of potato chips on the shelf. Help yourselves!", there would be a stampede to get to the shelf first. It is clear from these examples that inattentive listening occurs when the priorities of the participants are not the same.

Control is often an issue in communication and is the effect of feelings of inadequacy. It is a maneuver used to divert the communicative process away from emotionally charged or self-revealing data. Control is manifested in several ways, for example, the speaker can monopolize the conversation, forcing the listener into a silent passive role. This domineering sender has time for only his views, his opinions and his belief systems and therefore rarely pays attention to the receiver. Another method of control is via incessant, trivial and superfluous details that mask relevant messages. With this method the recipient is so deluged with issues and details that he cannot acknowledge, understand or interrupt the rapid flow of communication. A third way in which control is manifested is through the use of minimal verbal activity. In this instance the messages are short and often vague, providing the receiver with little understanding of either the message or its purpose. A fourth means of control used in the communication process is through the use of hackneyed words or phrases. The deployment of stock phrases keeps the level of communication on a superficial, uninvolved basis and conveys to the receiver a lack of genuine interest. How often have you met a friend or acquaintance who says to you, "Good Morning! How are you?" and continues on his way. He has accomplished a socially acceptable greeting but has not waited for your reply. Are you left with the impression that he is interested about what you think and feel?

The nurse must realize that not only patients try to exert these kinds of control. The therapeutic professional can also make interventive errors by exercising the same methods of control; the dynamics, however, differ in scope. The professional can control the therapeutic communicative process by remaining superficial, talking too much about generalities, or by focusing on secondary (background) data in order to avoid emotionally charged data. This error is a subconscious effort to mask a fear of therapeutic failure in effectively and successfully handling data with the patient.

3) inaccurate interpretations of message

Communicators must always remain conscious of the fact that perception is highly individualistic and that therefore it is relatively easy to fall into the communication traps of making generalizations, assumptions and in over-identifying. In these traps, the original intent is lost, and the receiver is left with the feeling that the message or the sender is not important enough to be heard and responded to appropriately.

To generalize is to form an illogical, exaggerated premise based on insufficient factual information. Generalization is the process by which a set of circumstances that are applicable in a majority of settings are applied indiscriminately to every set of circumstances without consideration for the "specific" differences which apply to an individual person's life experiences. To illustrate, here is an example of an actual incident.

> Miss Kane, a black student nurse, was assigned to give a patient, Mrs. Jones, a back rub. Mrs. Jones is an Appalachian who had recently moved to a large industrial city with her husband and three children. Her speech was still thick with the accent of her native area. Miss Kane observed that Mrs. Jones became rigid when she began the back rub; she interpreted this as a sign of Mrs. Jones' racial prejudice.
>
> In relating the incident to her classmates, Miss Kane stated that Mrs. Jones told her that she had never had a stranger bathe her or rub her back. Miss Kane had completely overlooked these comments as possibly significant causes for Mrs. Jones' tension.

An assumption is defined as attributing meaning to a message based on one's own frame of reference. Suppose a person says to you, "I'm going to take a rest." This comment can be interpreted in many ways. While to rest generally means to sit or to lie in a motionless position, we all know individuals who rest by pursuing an active hobby, exercising, taking a shower, paying a visit to the beauty shop or going for a drive in the country. To avoid the assumption trap and to interpret accurately, you must seek clarification of the communicated message. You must discover what "rest" means to that person. Neither the necessity for accurate interpretation nor the acknowledgement of a person's uniqueness of individual perception can be emphasized strongly enough. Just think about the popular gift books, ceramics or song entitled "Happiness is . . .," and you realize the many meanings the term implies! But remember—it has a particular significance for each individual person in a particular setting at a particular point in time.

Overidentification occurs when an individual hears what is being said and immediately interprets the message according to his own value systems or frames of reference. It occurs because what is being said may be similar to the listener's own experience. Accordingly, the listener either agrees, disagrees, approves, disapproves or in some other way makes a value judgment about the message or the sender. In other words, the listener "jumps to conclusions" and regards the conclusion he reaches as valid.

Making assumptions and overgeneralizations leads the receiver of the communicated message into responding with specific communication tactics. Some of the more common tactics are: stating his personal opinions as fact, giving a "pep talk," providing advice, offering "pat answers" for problems or offering false reassurance. In each of the preceding, self-worth, self-expression, uniqueness, individuality, concern, empathy and acceptance are all denied, and thoughtful consideration of the meaning and intent of the communicated message is by-passed. Objectivity and rationality are lost. The respondent does not hear with understanding; therefore, the communication exchange is terminated.

4) failure to maintain personal integrity

Communication is often abruptly terminated because the participants fail to be honest with themselves and with the person with whom they are communicating. Integrity is synonymous with honor. Personal integrity is based on the amount of respect one has for self which in turn influences the respect one is able to demonstrate toward another. Breaking promises, withholding information, giving misinformation or providing a too-detailed description or explanation are communication tactics which demonstrate a lack of personal integrity. Honesty within the communication process is suspect when promises are made and not kept. Giving one's verbal word is just as binding as signing one's name to a written contract. One should never make a promise one does not intend to keep. Nor should one withhold information to which another is legitimately entitled. A person has a right to know those facts which concern him and his particular situation or which might influence him to act in a particular way. It is not unusual to hear words like, "I'm not going to tell him, for his own good," or "What he doesn't know won't hurt him." These are false premises and are usually employed when the speaker is afraid to be "real" or is afraid that he will be called upon to accept responsibility for another's action or reaction. A person has a right to self-determination, that is, to decide for himself what is or what is not "good" for him.

Misinformation is often transmitted because the speaker lacks knowledge and attempts to save face by supplying any answer. What the speaker fails to realize is that giving misinformation is far more damaging to his projected image than an honest, open "I don't know." Self-respect can be enhanced by such an admission; misinformation can only tarnish it.

Communication barriers lead to dead ends. They cause misunderstanding, apprehension, anxiety and confusion for both sender and receiver. They are pitfalls that must be avoided at all costs. Learning to communicate is like learning to walk. First, you must be able to crawl, then to stand and hang on, and finally, you take your own independent steps. In those first steps, you feel like you are walking on eggs. Becoming skillful in the art of communication, like learning to walk, requires patience, practice, perserverance and determination.

effective therapeutic communication practices

Therapeutic communication, unlike social communication, is a goal-oriented, planned, purposeful pursuit. It is neither left to chance nor undertaken without thoughtful consideration and preparation. Before the nurse begins to implement the therapeutic nurse-patient relationship in an effective manner, she must become aware of specific communication practices and develop skill in the execution of these practices. We have devised three major categories into which communication practices may be divided. They are as follows.

I Practices Geared to Establishing a Climate for Communication

1 Select a setting that insures privacy and confidentiality.
2 Schedule and use the same setting for subsequent sessions.
3 Select a time which is mutually agreeable.
4 Assess and modify the environment to promote physical and psychological comfort.
5 Eliminate possible environmental and personal distractions.
6 Provide for appropriate seating.
7 Modify interpersonal spacing according to patient's and nurses' needs.
8 Explain time limits.
9 Modify length of interaction according to patient's tolerance for close, interpersonal contact.
10 Modify length of interaction based on patient's ability to concentrate.
11 Start and end session on time.
12 Contract with the patient for the method of recording the communication.
13 Assume a body posture that conveys interest, attention and respect.
14 Maintain an unbiased or friendly facial expression and attitude.
15 Speak with a clear, well-modulated tone of voice.
16 Maintain eye contact.

II Practices Geared to Developing Approaches to Facilitate Communication

    1 State the goals of the interaction.

    2 Allow and encourage the patient to assume the initiative in the interaction process.

    3 Encourage and support a free exchange of ideas, thoughts and feelings.

    4 Permit the patient to move at his own pace.

    5 Guide the interaction from the simple to the complex.

    6 Direct the focus of the communication on reality, on the patient and on his needs.

    7 Focus on problem areas.

    8 Send messages in a form the patient can understand.

    9 Send messages using language which has meaning for both nurse and patient.

    10 Send messages according to the patient's rate of ability to receive.

    11 Identify themes and recurring behaviors.

    12 Modify practice and technique according to the need of the patient.

III Practices Geared to Implementing a Verbal Exchange which Focuses on Specific Identifiable Skills

    1 Use indirect questions or comments to facilitate interaction.

    2 Use direct questions only when specific information is needed.

    3 Give short responses.

    4 Encourage the patient to elaborate.

    5 Reflect feelings or ideas.

    6 Note changes in subject matter.

    7 Identify and explore discrepancies between verbal and nonverbal behavior.

    8 Introduce new thoughts and ideas when the patient indicates readiness to hear, discuss or accept.

    9 Wait during silences.

    10 Use feedback to determine understanding of transmitted messages.

    11 Identify with the patient specific concerns regarding himself and his relationship with others.

    12 Summarize dialogue between participants.

    13 Explore each of the identified concerns through description and clarification.

    14 Compare and validate perceptions.

15 Extract from content, data for interpretation.

16 Formulate with the patient possible alternatives or solutions.

17 Support the patient in his attempt to test out the solutions.

18 Evaluate with the patient results of testing.

19 Identify strengths and weakness of the communication process within the interaction.

20 Assess the level of involvement of the participants in the interaction.

21 Evaluate the level of nurse-patient participation using as standards the principles for effective communication found on pages 25-28 and the stated goals of the interaction.

22 Write objectives for nursing care based on the interpretation of the evaluation.

23 Revise goals for subsequent interactions based on interpretations of evaluation.

24 Identify objectives for improving nurse effectiveness.

25 Keep an accurate record of the interaction.

therapeutic techniques of communication

Effective communication functioning within the nurse-patient relationship depends on an understanding of others and the process of communication. It also depends on the ability of the nurse to employ certain identified techniques of communication. These techniques are tools by which the nurse carries out communication practices. The tools are important only in the sense that they facilitate the communication process. The techniques are not meant to be memorized and used by the nurse as a stereotyped approach or response. In and of themselves, they are not absolutes, and their use does not guarantee therapeutic effectiveness. They are merely the means by which the nurse conveys her ability to be therapeutic. In order for the communication process to be therapeutic, the nurse must modify and adapt the techniques to the peculiarities of the participants and the prevailing situation.

The therapeutic techniques commonly employ questions as the usual method of operation. It is important for the nurse to remember that direct questions tend to decrease communication, and that indirect or open-ended questions are far more productive. In employing the skills of communication, the nurse should be careful to particularly avoid using those direct questions that illicit only a "yes" or "no" response as these types of questions produce no feedback and tend to create an inquisitional atmosphere. However, direct questions can and should be used when specific facts are needed. Broad openings and general leads are more appropriate in that they allow the patient to take the initiative as well as provide an opportunity for him to expand on the topics under discussion. Questioning leads, using "how and why," also require careful consideration in their application. Too many hows and whys tend to increase feelings of inadequacy when the patient's response comes back, "I don't know." A response to a how or why question requires that an individual is able to think in a rational, procedural, organized manner and realize causes and implications.

All questions should be clear and precise. The nurse must bear in mind that responses to questions are more dependent on the form the questions take rather than the person to whom the question is directed. In other words, if a question is not clear or precise, no person can be expected to respond appropriately. Therefore, the kind, the manner and the purpose of the question become significant factors in implementing the communication practices and applying the skills of communication.

In Table 3-1 we present nine common therapeutic techniques of communication. We identify the technique, define it, indicate its purpose and provide concrete examples to demonstrate its use.

TABLE 3-1
NINE COMMON THERAPEUTIC TECHNIQUES OF COMMUNICATION

Technique	Definition	Purpose	Examples
Exploring	Obtaining all pertinent data on a particular subject or feeling.	1) To increase the level of self-perception of the participants.	P: I feel sad about going but not so sad that I _____. N: What?
		2) To acquire mutually understood information.	P. I heard them talking about me in the hall. N. Tell me about the incident.
		3) To move beyond the superficial and deal with the more complex or hidden meanings of the message.	P: I don't feel well today. N: What seems to be the matter?
		4) To encourage the sender to evaluate described material.	P: I want to get married to a woman who is living with another man, but I don't know . . . N: You seem unsure—you don't know what?
Clarifying	Attempting to find the meaning of the communicated message.	1) To establish mutual understanding.	P: I have a pass to go home for the weekend. N: What does this mean to you?
		2) To identify common meanings associated with terms or phrases.	P: That nurse has pilot's eyes. N: What do you mean?
		3) To promote and encourage further communication between the participants.	P: Gone are days when things were simple. N: I'm not sure I understand what you are trying to tell me.
		4) To facilitate the recognition of individual differences.	

TABLE 3-1 (continued)

Technique	Definition	Purpose	Examples
		5) To decrease distortions in perception. 6) To decrease the level of verbal distortions.	
Reflecting	Conveying to the sender his expressed thoughts and related feelings.	1) To acknowledge to the sender that the message has been received. 2) To demonstrate to the sender that the receiver is searching for understanding of the message. 3. To enable the sender to perceive the communication as an extension of self. 4) To promote objectivity in determining the meaning of the message.	P: She just burns me up! N: You sound angry. P: I finished my O.T. project. Everyone thought it was pretty good. N: You seem pleased with yourself.
Focusing	Concentrating on a specific thought or feeling regarding a particular point.	1) To draw the attention of the sender to significant data. 2) To encourage the sender to separate relevant data from the irrelevant. 3) To sustain goal-oriented communication. 4) To discourage the sender from rambling. 5) To interrupt and forestall rapid subject changes.	P: Tom is always picking on me, no matter what I do. N: Give me an example. P: They said I can't go home. N: Who are "they"?
Informing	Responding to direct questions with needed facts.	1) To share knowledge. 2) To promote understanding. 3) To make facts clear. 4) To build trust.	P: What time do I go do the dentist? N: You have a 1:00 appointment. P: What about this information? Who gets to see it? N: Only me and my instructor.

TABLE 3-1 (continued)

Techniques	Definition	Purpose	Examples
		5) To establish confidence in and reliability of the sender.	
Using Silence	Communicating without verbalization.	1) To convey the receiver's interest, acceptance and understanding.	P: My mother has been saying that she does not want me home permanently. That's not a good feeling. N: (remains silent)
		2) To allow the sender to assume initiative.	P: They always got me out before. I'd love to go home, that's for sure. N: (remains silent)
		3) To provide the sender with time to collect and sort out his thoughts.	P: I hope she lets me return home. I'm scared. I don't know where I will live if I can't go home. N: (remains silent)
		4) To provide an opportunity to share with the sender his indirectly expressed feelings.	
		5) To emphasize a point.	
		6) To provide an opportunity to introduce a new idea or feeling.	
		7) To allow for relief from emotionally charged content.	
Validating	Confirming one's observations and interpretations.	1) To facilitate accurate appraisal of the sender and his communicated message.	P: I didn't want to come but my mother brought me anyhow! N: Sometimes it's difficult to do the things we have to do.
		2) To avoid making assumptions.	P: Yeah, they're always yelling at each other and at me. N: It must be hard to keep your cool when everybody is yelling.
		3) To verify cues.	
		4) To arrive at mutual understanding that increases rapport and establishes a basis for collaboration	

TABLE 3-1 (continued)

Techniques	Definition	Purpose	Examples
Evaluating	Assessing the significance of a communicated message.	1) To determine progress.	P: I am getting better. N: In what ways do you feel better?
		2) To acknowledge differences.	P: As a child my brother was always in the limelight. Everybody noticed him. N: It must have been very difficult for you. Can you recall how you felt then?
		3) To provide feedback from which clarification and understanding is derived.	
		4) To make comparisons and exercise judgment so that the sender is better able to engage in decision making.	
Summarizing	Developing a concise résumé of the communicated message.	1) To facilitate recall of important points.	P: That's all I have to say today. N: During the session you and I have discussed . . .
		2) To promote clarification and achieve new understandings.	(At the initiation of a session the nurse begins with summary of last session.) N: Last time we talked about some of your feelings about being here in the hospital . . .
		3) To maintain a point of interest.	
		4) To provide a basis for developing a plan of action.	
		5) To bring discussion of a particular subject to a conclusion.	

The following excerpts of data from nurse-patient interactions demonstrates the use of the therapeutic techniques of communication.

situation I

Danny, age 13, was referred for psychotherapy by Juvenile Court. His mother remained with Danny during the first session to provide the nurse with background information. On the second visit his mother stated that Danny was scared and wanted her to remain with him. During this second session Danny sat opposite the nurse, crossed his legs left over right, sat with his head down, playing with his shoe strings and avoiding looking directly at the nurse. For the most part, he did not verbally respond to the nurse's open-ended approaches. Periods of silence were breached by the mother.

Dialogue in Interaction	*Comments*
Nurse: Tell me something about yourself.	A general open-ended statement is used to elicit information, to put him at ease and to encourage him to assume the initiative.
(Danny gives a grunt that is followed by a pause which lasts one minute.)	
Mother, *(turns to Danny):* Danny, before we came you were telling me about cutting up at school and the bad influence of your friends and you wanted to know about changing schools.	
Danny: I just can't get Cs at W	
(Mother turns to nurse and talks about private schools versus public schools and says what she thinks should be done about Danny's schooling.)	Mother is aware of Danny's discomfort and even though she too is uneasy, she tries to protect him.
Nurse, *(interrupts mother, turns to Danny):* Danny, what do you think prevents you from getting Cs?	Direct question for focusing and exploring.
Danny: Too much fooling around!	
(Mother interjects a long explanation of the school schedule.)	
Nurse, *(turns to Danny's mother):* I'd like Danny and me to spend the rest of the time together getting to know each other. Would you mind waiting downstairs?	Clarifying the role of nurse therapist. Mother's presence inhibits the development of the therapeutic nurse-patient relationship.
(Mother hesitates, then nods her head and leaves the room.)	
Nurse: I asked your mother to leave because I thought you find it hard to talk with me while she was here.	
(Danny makes no verbal response.)	
Nurse, *(after pausing):* Danny, tell me more about yourself.	
(Danny makes no verbal response.)	
(Nurse waits 5 minutes.)	Silence used for the purpose of demonstrating interest and acceptance. Provides opportunity for Danny to assume the initiative.

Dialogue in Interaction	Comments
Nurse: It takes time for strangers to get to know each other, and communicating with adults might be difficult.	Informing to promote understanding.
(Danny avoids looking at the nurse, sits with head down and plays with pant legs and shoes. After waiting through 5 minutes of silence the nurse verbalizes her observations at two-minute intervals.)	
Nurse: You might be having trouble finding words to begin.	Reflecting to acknowledge to Danny that his behavior is understood.
(Danny grimaces.)	
Nurse: Perhaps you didn't want to come to see me, and that might be making you angry.	Reflecting and clarifying to promote continued understanding.
(Danny shows increased agitated movements.)	
Nurse: How do you feel about having to come for counseling?	Validating of impression. Direct question to draw attention to the connection between behavior, feelings and demands placed on him by the court.
(Danny shrugs his shoulders.)	
Nurse: An hour's session is a long time. I think it might help us to get better acquainted if we have two half-hour sessions per week.	Informing to encourage further communication. Evaluation to provide feedback.
(Danny shows no change in behavior.)	
Nurse: I'll contact Mr. S about your school schedule and let you know the response at the next session.	Informing to share plans for action.
(Still no change in Danny.)	
Nurse: Our time is up. I'll see you next Monday and Friday for a half hour.	Informing to promote understanding.
(Danny immediately runs out of the room)	

Danny missed his second appointment because he went to visit some friends and later told his parents that he forgot. At the third session, Danny reluctantly entered the office, selected a seat opposite the nurse and acknowledged her good morning with a "Hi!"

Dialogue in Interaction	Comments
Danny: What did Mr. S have to say?	It should be noted that while Danny did not verbally respond to the nurse in the previous session and even missed a session, he immediately initiated the interview by recalling an issue raised in the last session—a definite indication that though one may not think the patient is paying any attention, every word is heard and many are remembered!
Nurse: I called him but he was busy. I left a message for him to call me back. I'm waiting for his call now. If it doesn't come today I will call him again first thing in the morning.	Informing to share knowledge.
(Danny nods his head affirmatively.)	
Nurse: What did you think about the last session?	Encouraging evaluation to provide feedback.
Danny: What do you mean, what did I think?	
Nurse: What were some of your feelings about it?	Explaining to encourage Danny to take the initiative.
Danny: I'm tired. I didn't want to come today.	Danny changed the subject, apparently unable to verbalize feelings at this point. Danny remained silent for 10 minutes. Opening with, "I'm tired" is also an effort by the patient to avoid emotional content. Though it may not be necessary to pick up and discuss, the nurse must be consciously aware of what reasons might provoke this type of opening.
Nurse: Tell me something about school, what you like or dislike?	Redirecting focus to his initial concern.
Danny: Teachers are stupid. They yell at you.	
Nurse: Stupid? In what way? Give me some other examples in which you think teachers are stupid.	Reflecting and clarifying. Exploring.
Danny: When you cut study hall or your lunch period and they catch you.	
Nurse: How is that being stupid?	Clarifying.

	Dialogue in Interaction	Comments
Danny,	(shrugs shoulders): You gotta go to the office. Sometimes they don't do nothing.	
Nurse:	They don't say anything?	Reflecting.
Danny:	You have to go back to where you're supposed to be.	
Nurse:	And that's being stupid?	Validating.
Danny:	Yeah.	
Nurse:	It's sometimes hard to do the things you're suppoed to do.	Reflecting.
Danny,	(makes no response for approximately one minute): Nobody likes Mr. S.	
Nurse:	I wonder why?	Exploring.
Danny:	He makes you do things you have to do.	
Nurse:	Oh! I see.	Exploring.
Danny:	Nobody in the whole school likes him.	
Nurse:	That's an awful lot of people to have not liking you.	Evaluating.
(Danny is silent.)		
Nurse:	Do you dislike Mr. S too?	Focusing.
(More silence.)		
Nurse:	What else about school do you like or dislike?	Exploring and refocusing.
Danny:	Nothing!	
Nurse:	It's sometimes difficult to share feelings.	Verbalizing the implied.
Danny:	Yeah.	
Nurse:	Today you shared with me some thoughts you have about school. Perhaps in our next session we can talk more around your feelings.	Summarizing and setting up a plan of action for the next session.

situation II

This second excerpt is from an actual series of interactions that took place between a student nurse and a 40-year-old white male who was diagnosed as a schizophrenic, catatonic type. The illustration is extracted from the fifth interaction the student had with this patient.

Dialogue in Interaction	Comments
Mr. Wyle: What do you want to ask?	
Student: I don't want to ask anything, Mr. Wyle. Is there something you'd like to talk about?	Informing and explaining.
Mr. Wyle: There's not much to tell, like I told you before—about getting a lawyer—both my sisters say I don't take my medicine and that's how they got me into the hospital. And I say I do take my medicine. My whole family thinks I'm crazy and I don't. Otherwise, I couldn't carry on a conversation like this.	
Student: You're telling me that you and your lawyer are trying to prove that you are capable of handling your own affairs. Am I correct?	Validating.
Mr. Wyle: Yes, that's just about the size of it.	
Student: Okay, what would you say or what could you do to prove the point that you are capable of handling your own affairs?	Focusing. Exploring.
Mr. Wyle: Well, just prove it to certain people, like Dr. Kriss for one.	
Student: And you can do this by . . .	Exploring.
Mr. Wyle: Yeah, by taking my medicines.	
Student: Before, you told me that sometimes you forget. Then your behavior changes.	Validating.
Mr. Wyle: Naw—it don't change that much!	
Student: But it does some?	Validating.
Mr. Wyle: It doesn't change at all as far as I'm concerned.	
Student: At all?	Reflecting.
Mr. Wyle: Well, maybe some, but not that much to have me "stamped insane." What behavior would I have? I don't go around stealing and knocking people in the head!	
Student: You stated before that you forget what you do when you don't take your medicine.	Validating.
Mr. Wyle: Forget? I don't forget.	
Student: Wait a minute, Mr. Wyle. We seem to be getting off the track.	Focusing.

Dialogue in Interaction	Comments
Mr. Wyle: You mean take medicine and stuff?	
Student: And what happened when you forgot it?	Exploring.
Mr. Wyle: Not much! My mother used to complain.	
Student: Complain?	Reflecting.
Mr. Wyle: Yeah, about what I did.	
Student: What did you do?	Exploring.
Mr. Wyle: She's very old, you know, and sometimes she doesn't even notice if she's giving it to me or not.	
Student: And you don't remind her?	Reflecting.
Mr. Wyle: Well, I feel I'm a little bit too old to be guided along by her hand. After all she's 63. Personally, I hate to tell you this but I hate to be around her because she is so old. I have to realize that what she says half the time is from age.	
Student: Give me an example.	Exploring.
Mr. Wyle: Well like, she says "Why don't you own a car?" and I said, "I don't know. I don't have the money." She said, "I'll save the money for you." And I said, "But you don't give me the freedom that it takes to drive a car." 'Cause theoretically, being in a place like this you shouldn't be able to drive a car 'cause it "stamps" you as being mentally ill. Mentally ill people shouldn't be allowed to drive a car. How should they? And endanger lives of other people.	
Student: What do you mean by "stamped mentally ill?" That seems to upset you.	Focusing. Validating.
Mr. Wyle: Why sure it does! Because I'm not mentally ill.	
Student: Could you give me a definition of being mentally ill?	Clarifying
Mr. Wyle: Mentally ill?	
Student: Yes.	Informing.

Dialogue in Interaction	Comments
Mr. Wyle: A mentally ill person is a person that is sick, hears voices, that goes around talking to himself, that goes around doing oddball actions that the rest of society doesn't do . . . And has fits, and takes a catatonic fit.	
Student: Catatonic fit?	Clarifying.
Mr. Wyle: Yeah, you know, goes around like this (*he starts shaking, rolling his eyes and wriggling*) and hears voices.	
Student: Do you ever hear voices?	Exploring.
Mr. Wyle: No, but this guy in the group he hears voices. He's got a problem, he shouldn't drive a car or be in public working.	
Student: Do you have a problem?	Exploring.
Mr. Wyle: Yes, I got a problem—taking this medication. Now why does she have to inject it?	
Student: We discussed this last week, Mr. Wyle. We decided that you would have to discuss receiving injections with Dr. Kriss.	Informing.
Mr. Wyle: Yeah, that's right. (*He rolls his eyes back.*)	
Student: What were you thinking about just now?	Reflecting.
Mr. Wyle: I was just wondering if I asked you, if you heard voices, would you tell me you heard them?	
Student: Now that I know you, yes, I would tell you.	Informing.
Mr. Wyle: Well you're honest. I see you're honest. I'll have to think about . . . (*seemed to be concentrating*)	
(*Silence for 2 minutes.*)	Using silence.
Mr. Wyle: So what you said you would risk being "stamped mentally ill" and tell someone that you heard voices, in order that they may help you understand why you heard them.	
Student: Yes, Mr. Wyle—that is what I mean.	Validating.
Mr. Wyle: Hmm!	

Dialogue in Interaction	Comments
Student: Mr. Wyle it's almost time to end the interview for today. We talked about several things, mainly your concern about being labeled mentally ill, taking your medication, some difficulties with your mother and about people hearing voices. Next time let's talk about some of these things in more detail.	Summarizing

situation III

Miss Smythe is a 43-year-old white female who was admitted to a medical floor with the diagnosis of a cerebral vascular accident. She is a Catholic, and shortly after admission, the hospital chaplain visited her and administered while she was unconscious the Sacrament of the Sick, "Last Rites." When Miss Smythe regained consciousness and was informed she became exceedingly angry and refused to see the chaplain again. She was very concerned about her care and frequently talked about leaving the hospital, but at the same time refused to participate in her care. A student was assigned to care for Miss Smythe. The following dialogue took place during morning care.

Dialogue in Interaction	Comments
Nurse: Good morning, Miss Smythe, my name is Miss Rosario and I will be caring for you this morning.	Giving information. Stating purpose.
Miss Smythe: Rosario, Rosario, that's Italian isn't it? You're a Catholic, aren't you? I'm a Catholic, too. Do you know what the church did to me? They gave me the Last Rites. I'm dead already and I don't know it. They knew it!	
Nurse: You really seem upset this morning.	Reflection of feeling.
Miss Smythe: Yes! Yes, I am! You'd be upset too if they did that to you.	
Nurse: Tell me more about what's been happening.	Exploring to encourage verbalization of feeling.
Miss Smythe: I told you! They gave me the Sacrament of the Dead while I was unconscious.	

Dialogue in Interaction		Comments
Nurse:	The Sacrament of the Dead? I'm not sure what you mean.	Asking for clarification.
Miss Smythe:	You know, the last Sacrament they give you when you're dying. I'm not dead yet.	
Nurse:	The fact that you received the Sacrament must have been very frightening.	Validating impression.
(Miss Smythe begins to cry.)		
(Nurse moves chair to bedside, sits down and remains with patient as she cries.)		Using silence.

As a result of this outburst, the relief experienced through the tears, the support provided by the nurse's presence, and the opportunity to further verbalize and explore feelings, the patient was able to come to a better understanding of her condition. She was able to ask questions about the amount of residual paralysis, the extent of disability she could expect and if the limitations would prevent her from returning to her job.

In this chapter we have highlighted the basics of the communicative process and illustrated some of the therapeutic techniques. Some of it is skeletal; we have deliberately eliminated details, expansion of concepts and thorough dialogues. The reader is referred to other references that explain the dynamics of communication and the therapeutic processes in depth. However, this chapter on the method, practice and process of communications offers the essential components that help the nurse develop her communicative skills in mental health practice.

suggested readings

Ball, Geraldine. "Speaking Without Words." *American Journal of Nursing,* Vol. 60 No. 5 (May, 1960), 692-693.

Barbara, Dominick A. *The Art of Listening.* Charles C. Thomas: Springfield, Illinois, 1966.

Barker, Larry, and Kibler, Robert J., eds. *Speech Communication Behavior: Perspective and Principles.* Prentice-Hall, Inc.: Englewood Cliffs, New Jersey, 1971.

Barnlund Dean C. *Interpersonal Communication—Survey and Studies.* Houghton Mifflin Co.: New York, 1968.

Benjamin, Alfred. *The Helping Interview.* 2d ed. Houghton Mifflin Co.: Boston, 1969.

Bermosk, Loretta Sue, and Mordan, Mary Jane. *Interviewing in Nursing.* MacMillan Co.: New York, 1964.

Blondis, Marion Nesbitt, and Jackson, Barbara E. *Nonverbal Communication with Patients: Back to the Human Touch.* John Wiley and Sons: New York, 1977.

Collins, Mattie. *Communication in Health Care.* C. V. Mosby Co.: St. Louis, 1977.

Cosper, Bonnie. "How Well Do Patients Understand Hospital Jargon?" *American Journal of Nursing,* Vol. 77 No. 12 (December, 1977), 1932-1934.

Dahl, Barbara W. "Formality Versus Familiarity: Communicating With Names." *Ohio Nurses Review,* LIII, No. 4 (April, 1978), 5-6.

Davis, Anne J. "The Skills Of Communication." *American Journal of Nursing,* Vol. 63 No. 1 (January, 1963), 66-70.

Eldred, Stanley H. "Improving Nurse-Patient Communication." *American Journal of Nursing,* Vol. 60 No. 11 (November, 1960), 1600-1602.

Fast, Julius. *Body Language.* M. Evans and Company, Inc.: New York, 1970.

Goldin, Phyllis, and Russell, Barbara. "Therapeutic Communication." *American Journal of Nursing,* Vol. 69 No. 9 (September, 1969), 1928-1930.

Greenhill, Maurice H. "Interviewing with a Purpose." *American Journal of Nursing,* Vol. 56 No. 10 (October 1956), 1259-1267.

Hall, Edward T. The Silent Language. Fawcett: Connecticut, 1959.

Hays, Joyce S., and Larson, Kenneth. *Interacting With Patients.* Macmillan Co.: New York, 1963.

Hein, Eleanor C. *Communication in Nursing Practice.* Little, Brown and Co.: Boston, 1973.

Hewitt, Helen E., and Pesznecker, Betty L. "Blocks to Communicating with Patients." American Journal of Nursing, Vol. 64 No. 7 (July, 1964), 101-103.

Hood, Mabel, "You Don't Always Need To Communicate." *Nursing Care* (August, 1977), 28.

Kesler, Arlene Riley. "Pitfalls To Avoid in Interviewing Outpatients." *Nursing 77,* Vol. 7 No. 9 (September, 1977), 70-73.

Kron, Thora. *Communication in Nursing.* W. B. Saunders Company: Philadelphia, 1967.

Lewis, Garland K. *Nurse-Patient Communication.* Wm. C. Brown Co.: Dubuque, Iowa, 1969.

Mercer, Lianne S., and O'Connor, Patricia. *Fundamental Skills In The Nurse-Patient Relationship: A Programmed Text.* W. B. Saunders Co.: Philadelphia, 1974.

Miller, George A., ed. *Communication, Language and Meaning: Psychological Perspectives.* Basic Books: New York, 1973.

O'Brien, Maureen J. *Communications and Relationships in Nursing.* C.V. Mosby Co.: St. Louis, 1974.

Orem, Dorothea E. *Nursing: Concepts of Practice.* McGraw-Hill Book Company: New York, 1971.

Orlando, Ida Jean. *The Dynamic Nurse-Patient Relationship.* G. P. Putnam and Sons: New York, 1961.

Paton, Margaret M. "I Told Them All." *American Journal of Nursing,* Vol. 76 No. 1 (January, 1976), 113.

Peplau, Hildegard. *Interpersonal Relations in Nursing.* Putnam Publishers: New York, 1952.

Peplau. Hildegard E. "Talking With Patients." *American Journal of Nursing*, Vol. 60 No. 7 (July, 1960), 964-966.

Pluckhan, Margaret L. *Human Communication: The Matrix of Nursing.* McGraw Hill Book Company: New York, 1978.

Reusch, Jurgen, and Bateson, Gregory. *Communication The Social Matrix of Psychiatry.* Norton and Co.: New York, 1968.

Robinson, Alice M. "Graffiti: Way-out Outlet for Patients." *R.N.,* Vol. 37 No. 1 (January, 1974), 38-39.

Scheflen, Albert E. *How Behavior Means.* Jason Aronson: New York, 1974.

Smith, Elaine. "Are You Really Communicating." *American Journal of Nursing,* Vol. 77 No. 12 (December, 1977), 1966-1968.

Smith, Virginia Whitmore. "I Can't Believe I Said That." *Nursing Outlook,* Vol. 18 No. 5 (May 1970), 51.

Sullivan, Harry Stark. *The Psychiatric Interview.* W. W. Norton and Co., Inc.: New York, 1954.

Thayer, Lee. *Communication and Communication Systems.* Richard D. Irwin, Inc.: Homewood, Illinois, 1968.

Travelbee, Joyce. *Interpersonal Aspects of Nursing.* F.A. Davis Co.: Philadelphia, 1966.

VanDersal, William. "How to Be a Good Communicator—And a Better Nurse." *Nursing 74* (December, 1974), 57-64.

Veninga, Robert. "Communications: A Patient's Eye View." *American Journal of Nursing.* Vol. 73 No. 2 (February, 1973), 320-322.

Wildhaber, Anita R. "The Silent Patients Speak." *R.N.,* Vol. 36 No. 5 (May, 1973), 108.

listen

When I ask you to listen to me
  and you start giving advice
  you have not done what I asked.

When I ask you to listen to me
  and you begin to tell me why I shouldn't feel that way,
  you are trampling on my *feelings*.

When I ask you to listen to me
  and you feel you have to *do* something to solve my problem,
  and you have failed me, strange as that may seem.

Listen! All I asked, was that you listen.
  not talk or do—just hear me.
Advice is cheap: 10 cents will get you both Dear Abby and
  Billy Graham in the same newspaper.
And I can do for myself; I'm not helpless.
  Maybe discouraged and faltering, but not helpless.

When you do something for me *that I can and need to do
for myself,* you contribute to my fear and weakness.

But, when you accept as a simple fact that I do feel what I feel,
  no matter how irrational, then I can quit trying to convince
  you and can get about the business of understanding what's
  behind this irrational feeling.
  And when that's clear, the answers are obvious and I
  don't need advice.
Irrational feelings make sense when we understand what's
  behind them.

Perhaps that's why prayer works, sometimes, for some people
  because God is mute, and he doesn't give advice or
  try to fix things. "They" just listen and let you
  work it out for yourself.

So, please listen and just hear me. And, if you want to
  talk, wait a minute for your turn; and I'll listen to you.

Anonymous

chapter 4

interpersonal relationships: a frame of reference

learning objectives

On completion of this chapter the reader should be able to:

1 Understand the term *relationship*.
2 Define *individual* and *group interpersonal relationships*.
3 Differentiate between *individual* and *group* relationships.
4 Have a basic comprehension of individual and group relationships within the context of the process of human development.

definition of terms

A simple definition of *relationship* is the existence of a connection or association between people. An *interpersonal relationship* is that relationship established between a person and those with whom the individual comes in contact, either on a one-to-one basis or in groups. There are various types of interpersonal relationships. First, there is the close, intimate contact with a "significant other." In this type of relationship, the significant other is that person with whom there has been established a reciprocal investment and on whom the individual relies for gratification of his interpersonal needs for affection, recognition and control. In other words, this close, intimate relationship involves a great deal of responsibility on the part of at least one of the individuals. This type of relationship is usually found between a parent and a child or a husband and a wife. It may also extend beyond the home to a relationship developed between close friends: a student and his teacher, a clergyman and his parishioner, or a nurse and her patient.

A second type of individual interpersonal relationship is one that is formed for specific goal-oriented purposes and supplementary need gratification. Specific goal-oriented purposes include such things as maintenance of lines of communication among family members, achievement of family concerns, carrying out cultural traditions and maintaining satisfactory work situations. Supplementary need gratification includes such things as meeting the basic human need for identification, belonging and security. This type of individual interpersonal relationship might be with a peer, a blood relation, an extended family member, an employer or a coworker.

A third type is one in which there are daily contacts between and among individuals whose significance may not be essential for daily living experiences and yet whose contact is necessary to further goal-directed activity. This type of individual interpersonal relationship is one that might be established with the check-out girl in the grocery store, with the mailman or with the next door neighbor. These particular relationships tend to preserve harmony and provide the "extras" in life.

Transactions within groups satisfy a person's need for establishing and maintaining his interdependency within the social, cultural and economic environments. As we have advanced in our technological development so too have our interdependent needs expanded within these environs. History reveals, with each era, shifts in the priorities of needs that affect interpersonal relationships—to man, with one or several others and with our environment. The twentieth century is an era of complex interdependent relationships. This complexity is manifested through the types of group relationships that individuals form.

Group relationships are divided into three major categories—primary, secondary and tertiary. The rationale for this categorization is based on the individual's need to set priorities in his search for fulfillment.

A *primary group* can be defined as a unit composed of close-knit, mutually interdependent and reciprocal memberships. In other words, the primary group is any small group to which an individual belongs because of a vested interest, specialized activity or fulfillment of need gratification. Familial, peer or religious groups are examples of primary groups. It is in conjunction with the primary group that the individual establishes the norms and mores for his particular position in life. It is through his continuous involvement with this type of group relationship that the individual finds validation for his ideas, thoughts, actions and feelings. This type of group relationship provides the members with group security and a means of identity, establishes role expectations and functionings and contributes a sense of belonging and acceptance.

Secondary groups are those formed for the purpose of enrichment and refinement of the individual's total living experience. The kinds of interdependent relationships formed within this category manifest a moderate degree of intimacy. The individual retains freedom to move in and out of secondary groups as his priorities change. This freedom of movement is unique to secondary groups and is another characteristic that distinguishes it from the primary group. A work group, a social club, an art class, or a professional organization exemplifies this secondary group category. Secondary group memberships are formed because they serve as a necessary and significant vehicle for the individual to meet his social, cultural and financial needs.

Tertiary groups are those in which there exists between members a limited degree of intimacy and involvement. Membership is based on the necessity for gratifying immediate needs. The relationships formed within the group are not designed to be continuous. They are based on priorities which, most likely but not exclusively, have been established by the individual within his primary or secondary groups. Participating in a fund raising campaign, becoming a member of a committee, joining a vacation tour group or taking part in a community action group is identified as a tertiary type of interpersonal group relationship.

development and progression of interpersonal relationships

Interpersonal relationships are learned experiences. They begin with birth and continue to deepen throughout the individual's life. Indelibly linked with the development of interpersonal relationships is the development of an individual's ability to communicate. For example, at birth an infant cries to announce its presence and to make known its needs. During infancy, the cry is the primary mechanism of communication between the infant and his world. The kind of response the infant receives from the mother or mother-substitute sets up a series of expectations on the part of the infant. These expectations may become habitual and lead to a specific pattern for the development of future interpersonal relationships.

In developing an interpersonal relationship there is a need for clarity and directness. A young child uses simple, direct language in interpersonal relationships that leaves little room for misinterpretation. Later interpersonal relationships are affected by the introduction of language complexities. The meanings of specific words and phrases take on varying colorations and connotations resulting in a gap between the sender and the receiver. This gap makes messages unclear and needs unheard. The individual at this point must constantly strive toward sustaining an interpersonal relationship by varying responses until the communication is clear and the message is heard and understood.

The development of interpersonal relationships is influenced by two other components found within the communication process: honesty and openness. Honesty in communications implies that the individual says what he means, what he thinks and what he feels. In early childhood the simple, direct communication reflects this honesty and openness. However, as the child grows, the continuation of this kind of forthright communication is often modified by the restraints society imposes for diplomacy and tact. These limitations are often confusing to the child. As a result he relinquishes a portion of his ability to be honest as a defensive protection for maintaining existing individual and group interpersonal relationships. The older the child grows, the more he uses lying, manipulating and storytelling. Honesty in communication is affected by the transactions within the child's systems of relationships. The more measurable degree of pathology within the child's relationship systems, the more he will use verbal games.

Openness refers to the individual's ability to communicate what he thinks and feels without fear of censure, ridicule or retaliation. This openness is again displayed in the child by direct and clear communication. Childlike openness is enhanced or inhibited by familial interactions and the way the primary group teaches the child to send messages—by positive example, by restricting openness through disciplinary action, rejection and failure to hear the messages or by using verbal corrections or subtle nonverbal innuendoes. Both the honesty and openness of the communication in early childhood is directly related to the degree to which trust and security have been demonstrated from his earliest interpersonal encounters.

Openness, like honesty, tends to decrease as communication complexity increases. The individual learns that openness leads to interpersonal risk and exposure of self. Feeling threatened, the individual communicates his thoughts and feelings more subtly in order to protect his present and future interpersonal associations. An individual's interpersonal relationships may appear satisfactory, but what does the individual do to himself in the process? Are the resultant relationships true? Are they significant? Meaningful? For some individuals, the answers to these questions are yes! For many others, the answers are no.

Generally, the natural components of communication—clarity, directness, honesty, and openness—contribute to and enhance an individual's relationship(s) with others. However, through the phases of growth and development and through the limitations imposed or perceived as imposed by society, an individual may sometimes sacrifice the naturalness of communication to preserve relationships. This is where the other components which influence interpersonal relationships come into play, that is, the perception of self in relation to the psycho-social and cultural factors influencing the developmental process. There is more to living than mere survival. During infancy, the mother-child relationship is markedly one-sided. Because the infant is totally dependent on others to meet his life sustaining needs, he identifies with and conforms to the expectations of those most important to him. The attitudes, feelings and behavior of individuals within the child's environment exert a strong influence on him and his relationship with others. Prevailing values of and attitudes toward such socio-cultural factors as the concepts of morality, humanity and sexuality; the norms for living, loving, learning, working, praying and playing; the expectations regarding success and failure; and the discrepancies in social sanctions—all become part of the developing self.

As the child progresses from a dependent state toward a state of independence and finally interdependence, the self emerges as a separate identity. Exposure to and involvement with significant others aids him in the search for this self. The individual struggles to identify, evaluate, retain or reject those attitudes and values which contribute to a feeling of wholeness or oneness with self. The maturation process is gradual and allows for the child to develop a realization of the "individual self" that becomes unique and different for every individual.

Interpersonal relationships are an end as well as a means toward reaching maturity. As a means to an end, they enhance perception of self. They alter perception of self, and they contribute to the continuous modification of self, thereby producing a "dynamic self." As an end, interpersonal relationships are a combined demonstration of the individual's acquired ability and skill both to communicate and to formulate a set of values and attitudes.

suggested readings

Ackerman, Nathan W. *The Psychodynamics of Family Therapy.* Basic Books, Inc.: New York 1958.

Brammer, Lawrence M., and Shostrom, Everett E. *Therapeutic Psychology.* Prentice-Hall, Inc.: Englewood Cliffs, New Jersey, 1968.

Brandner, Patty. "Women in Groups." *American Journal of Nursing*, Vol. 74 No. 9 (September, 1974), 1661-1664.

Burton, Genevieve. *Personal, Impersonal and Interpersonal Relations.* Springer: New York, 1964.

Downs, Florence S. "Technological Advances and The Nurse Family Relationships." *Nursing Digest*, Vol. 3 No. 3 (May/June, 1975), 23-24.

Fagin, Claire M. "Psychotherapeutic Nursing." *American Journal of Nursing*, Vol. 67 No. 2 (February, 1967), 298-304.

Heider, Fritz. *The Psychology of Interpersonal Relations.* John Wiley & Sons, Inc.: New York, 1958.

Lair, Jess. *"I ain't much, baby—but I'm all I've got."* Fawcett Publications, Inc.: Greenwich, Conn. 1974.

Sullivan, Harry Stack. *The Interpersonal Theory of Psychiatry.* W. W. Norton Co.: 1953.

chapter 5

the therapeutic use of self

learning objectives

On completion of this chapter the reader should be able to:

1 Define the *nurse-patient relationship*.
2 State the purpose and importance of the nurse-patient relationship.
3 Identify the basic concepts which are prerequistes for the successful achievement of the therapeutic goal.
4 Define and distinguish *love*, *empathy*, *sympathy*, *understanding* and *acceptance* in the nurse-patient relationship.

basic concepts identified

In nursing, interpersonal relationships take on an added significance primarily because nurses use the interpersonal process as the major tool to assist the patient in maintaining or restoring an optimal level of health, and preventing illness. Every encounter the nurse has with a patient, no matter how brief or for whatever purpose, should be used to either establish or maintain a nurse-patient relationship. The *nurse-patient relationship* is a therapeutic alliance. It is a transactional encounter. It is a goal-oriented, educative event that occurs between the patient and the nurse. The specific purpose of the relationship is to foster gradual changes through a series of events designed to help the patient deal with current reality, problems, needs, crises and encourage a process of resolution.

The implementation of and engagement in a nurse-patient relationship involves certain specific basic concepts. These basic concepts are love, empathy, sympathy, understanding and acceptance. The nurse's use of these basic concepts permits the establishment of rapport between herself and her patients. They are prerequisites to achieving therapeutic goals. These essential elements that the nurse must bring with her to the relationship are acquired through her professional educational and her personal growth. To what degree is the nurse expected to use these elements in the relationship? This depends on two factors: 1) the actual identified needs of the patient and 2) the ability of the nurse to help the patient meet his needs.

basic concepts defined

Love is a demonstration of care toward another human being. It is the basis of the nurse-patient relationship; without love a meaningful relationship cannot be formed. *To care* is to commit one's self, to invest one's time, effort and knowledge, to utilize specific skills born out of a willingness to help, to desire to share one's therapeutic self with another in problem solving and to be willing to become involved during stress and discomfort. *To be concerned* is to demonstrate respect for the individual as an unique human being, to acknowledge his intrinsic worth, and through one's behavior convey interest, compassion, warmth and comfort to the patient. When the nurse expresses care and concern the patient experiences a sense of self-worth, belonging, security and hope. Thereby the seeds of trust are sown. Unless the nurse achieves this level of interaction with the patient, movement toward the goals of a therapeutic relationship cannot be accomplished.

Nursing actions which convey this concept of love to the patient range from the very simple, as in the extension of common courtesies, to the very complex, as in the skillful application of a body of knowledge to practice. Some examples of simple activities include: a smile and nod of the head in greeting; addressing or referring to a person by name; apologizing when appropriate; supplying correct and necessary information and responding truthfully to questions. More complex activities include: attending to individual likes and dislikes; taking time to explain and to repeat explanations if need be; listening to a story told for the tenth time; providing an extra pillow or blanket; opening or closing a window; and being gentle or firm as appropriate. Nursing actions demonstrating an even greater degree of complexity might be: seeking the patient's collaboration in establishing mutually desired goals; keeping promises; insuring privacy; setting realistic expectations for patient behavior and repeatedly approaching the patient despite continuous rejection. The nurse can find many other ways to express love as she engages in the daily routine of the ward and treatment regimes. When done with love, the routines become therapeutic.

In nursing literature much confusion exists regarding the concepts of *empathy* and *sympathy*. Although these concepts, so essential to good nursing, have been used interchangeably, they are actually different. In order to distinguish between them, let us first look at the theories of the behavioral sciences and then at how nursing views and employs them in practice. In the behavioral sciences empathy is regarded as an essential tool of the therapeutic self. It enhances the ability of the therapist to fully grasp and comprehend the emotional tones of the patient in crisis. *Empathy* is a sustained quality of objective feeling. As a component of the nurse-patient relationship, it is the ability on the part of the nurse to feel "with" and "for" the patient. Its use requires that the nurse be able to set aside her own values, opinions and judgments and "see" the situation as it appears to the patient.

Empathy permits the nurse to increase her understanding of patient behavior by allowing her to identify the feeling states of the patient. This enables the nurse to support the patient and assist him in finding meaning in each of his experiences. To be empathetic does not necessarily require that the nurse has had a similar problem or crisis. The nurse must be aware that empathizing with the patient does not lead to internalizing his feelings. If internalization occurs the nurse has overidentified with the patient and has consequently decreased her nursing effectiveness.

The following case incident illustrates the concept of empathy in nursing practice.

> On a medical unit in Centerville General Hospital, the night nursing staff reported that Mr. Wilson was up at frequent intervals during the night and would often roam the corridors looking about with a scrutinizing eye. When approached by the night staff and told to return to his room he would grumble and say "Just leave me alone. I'm OK," or when offered a sleeping pill he would say, "Never take the stuff." The day staff complained of him as a "problem patient" because he spent the day sleeping. One night Miss Norton, a relief night nurse, found Mr. Wilson wandering the hospital corridor and instead of reporting him she took the patient into the nursing station to talk with him. During this conversation, Mr. Wilson revealed that, although retired, he had been a night watchman for 30 years and had spent daylight hours sleeping. He also stated that he had never broken this pattern and, even now, did much of his household work at night.

Miss Norton's use of empathy with this patient allowed her to understand the patient's behavior and to identify his feelings as opposed to applying personal views, values, opinions and judgments which would have resulted in the patient continuing to be labeled as a "problem." A prerequisite for the effective use of empathy is that the nurse have a clear understanding of herself and how she operates. The nurse with empathy exudes an aura of continued concern, interest, tolerance, and support.

Sympathy is regarded by the behavioral sciences as an element that can lead to detrimental outcomes of the therapeutic process through the loss of objectivity and countertransferences, i.e., the therapist's assumption of pseudopower and pseudocharacteristics as projected by the patient. Nevertheless, the nursing profession views sympathy as a therapeutic concept. Sympathy refers to a momentary feeling and the resultant action triggered by a specific situation. A display of sympathy on the part of the nurse is a recognition of the discomfort, pain or distress experienced by the patient. This recognition evokes an immediate response in the nurse to alleviate the condition. The application of sympathy to patient care is appropriate and needed. The nurse must exercise judgment in the application of sympathy and take precautions to prevent sympathy from turning into pity. Pity is inappropriate because it reduces nursing care to an ineffective level by decreasing the patient's self-worth, rendering the nurse equally helpless with the patient through overidentification, and lastly, producing dehumanization because the patient wants help rather than wanting to inflict suffering on another.

Understanding is both an intellectual function as well as a feeling state. As an intellectual function, understanding is a cultivated ability in which an individual demonstrates an awareness of the many subtle differences which influence a person and the development of his thoughts, feelings and actions. The affective or feeling state of understanding is the ability of the nurse to be aware of and show appreciation for another's thoughts, feelings and actions. This awareness and appreciation is demonstrated when the nurse views the patient as an individual and recognizes his uniqueness by selecting those specific nursing actions which best meet his needs.

The degree of understanding the nurse can achieve depends on her ability to love, to empathize and to sympathize with her patients. The nurse conveys understanding by listening attentively to her patients; learning about his uniqueness (cultural, religious, social, familial); maintaining a nonjudgmental attitude; extending warmth and kindness; seeking clarification of his communications and seeking validation for her interpretations. The nurse must exert a continuous, conscious effort to achieve this level of understanding.

Acceptance is an attitude of positive recognition and respect for a person. It is the last component needed by the nurse to promote a therapeutic interpersonal relationship and is, perhaps, the most difficult to achieve. An intellectual acknowledgement of acceptance is not enough. It must be accompanied by the emotional state of acceptance as demonstrated through an attitudinal change. It is the reception of an individual's pleasant and unpleasant ideas, emotions and behavior without censure or retaliation. Acceptance is recognition that the verbal and nonverbal communications expressed in any specific living experience is the outcome of an individual's total development and is, most likely, the best coping method he is able to demonstrate at that point. Acceptance does not imply agreement, approval or tolerance. The nurse demonstrates acceptance by supporting and encouraging the individual's efforts to satisfy his needs. Acceptance makes explicit the use of a basic principle in health care: to begin where the patient is and to make use of his potential capabilities to achieve an optimal level of functioning.

The basic concepts of love, empathy, sympathy, understanding and acceptance that the nurse nurtures and demonstrates toward her patient enables her to engage in a therapeutic interpersonal relationship either on an individual or group basis. These concepts are more than elements of personality; they are, in fact, a necessary part of nursing activity.

suggested readings

Barbieri, Winnie Kender. "No Pity." *American Journal of Nursing*, Vol. 76 No. 9 (September, 1976), 1482.

Carkhuff, Robert. *Helping and Human Relationships—A Primer For Lay and Professional Helpers*, Vols. I and II, Holt, Rinehart and Winston: New York, 1969.

Ehmann, Virginia E. "Empathy: its origin, characteristics and process." *Perspectives in Psychiatric Care*, Vol. 9 No. 2 (March-April, 1971), 72-80.

Fromm, Erich. *The Art of Loving*. Harper and Row: New York, 1956.

Glasser, William. *Reality Therapy*. Harper & Row: New York, 1965.

Haber, Judith, et al. *Comprehensive Psychiatric Nursing*. McGraw-Hill, Inc.: New York, 1978.

Hein, Eleanor, and Leavitt, Maribelle. "Providing Emotional Support to Patients." *Nursing 77,* Vol. 7 No. 5 (May, 1977), 38-41.

Kalisch, Beatrice J. "What is Empathy." *American Journal of Nursing*, Vol. 73 No. 9 (September, 1973), 1548-1552.

MacDonald, Malcolm R. "How Do Men and Women Students Rate in Empathy." *American Journal of Nursing*, Vol. 77 No. 6 (June, 1977), 998.

Older, Jules. "Four Taboos That May Limit the Success of Psychotherapy." *Psychiatry*, Vol. 40 (August, 1977), 197-204.

Peitchinins, Jacquelyn A. "Therapeutic Effectiveness of Counseling by Nursing Personnel: Review of the Literature." *Nursing Research*, Vol. 21 (March-April, 1972), 138-148.

Pluckhan, Margaret L. *Human Communication the Matrix of Nursing*. McGraw Hill Book Company: New York, 1978.

Rogers, Carl. *Client Centered Therapy*. Houghton-Mifflin Co.: Boston, 1951.

Schwartz, Morris S., and Schockley, Emmy Lanning. *The Nurse and the Mental Patient*. John Wiley & Sons, Inc.: New York, 1956.

Shanken, William J., and Shanken, Phyllis. "How To Be A Helping Person." *Journal of Psychiatric Nursing and Mental Health Services*, Vol. 14 No. 2 (February, 1976), 24-28.

Wilkiemeyer, Diana S. "Affection: Key to Care for the Elderly." *American Journal of Nursing*, Vol. 72 No. 12 (December, 1972), 2166-2168.

chapter 6

the therapeutic
nurse-patient relationship

learning objectives

On completion of this chapter the reader should be able to:

1 Understand *rapport* as the core concept in the establishment, development and maintenance of a therapeutic nurse-patient relationship.
2 Identify strategies which facilitate the interaction process.
3 Distinguish among the strategies of building trust, acknowledging and exploiting readiness and setting limits.
4 Become familiar with specific nursing activity which demonstrates the implementation of these strageties.
5 Describe the operational phases within the nurse-patient relationship process.
6 Identify the therapeutic tasks to be accomplished within the orienting, working and terminating phases of the nurse-patient relationship.
7 Recognize impediments to the nurse-patient relationship.
8 Recognize and implement specific intervention directed toward success in the therapeutic nurse-patient relationship.

69

the core concept

The crux of the therapeutic relationship is the systematic building of rapport. The achievement of rapport is the initial step toward an effective working therapeutic relationship. Rapport is a multifaceted core concept. It is:

A mutual sharing of the participants' humaneness.

A willingness to become involved with another person.

An openness which permits another person "to be" without inflicting penalty "for being."

A demonstration of a receptivity which intensifies the awareness of the participants' perceptions.

Growth toward mutual acceptance and understanding of individuality.

The end result of one's care and concern for another—in action.

Rapport is not a tangible substance, but it can be observed and felt. Rapport is that which leads to an atmosphere of mutual confidence. It can only be achieved when the nurse utilizes the above prerequisites of the therapeutic relationship and adopts a humanistic and holistic approach to life and living. The responsibility for initiation of rapport within the therapeutic relationship must be assumed by the nurse.

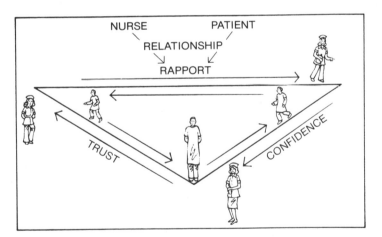

Figure 6-1

strategies

To facilitate the interaction process, the nurse must employ specific strategies. These strategies are designed to promote nurse-patient effectiveness as evidenced by the achievement of the mutually established goals of the relationship. They include building trust, acknowledging and utilizing readiness and setting limits.

building trust

Trust and rapport go hand in hand, but trust is not necessarily a direct result of rapport. One can achieve rapport without ever achieving trust. However in the therapeutic relationship, as the nurse develops rapport, she lays the foundation for building trust.

To trust is to believe in self and to believe in others. It implies that an individual can rely on himself or on another in all kinds of circumstances. In a relationship trust is a mutual exchange of faith. It allows for the acceptance of another's judgment as a possible means of attaining personal satisfaction through goal achievement or problem solving. Trust occurs in different degrees and is frequently tested by the participants in interpersonal encounters. Trust is an outgrowth of a feeling of security and is evidenced by respect for life. It is also evidenced by an awareness of life and a "zest for living." It is built on faith, hope and integrity.

The building of trust involves the use of a two-phase strategy. The first phase concerns the demonstration of the nurse's confidence in self. Her confidence is in direct proportion to her personal and professional knowledge and her ability to function as an integrated person. The nurse's self-confidence is demonstrated through the presentation of the "real self" rather than the presentation of an assumed "nursing role."

The second phase is concerned with the nurse's helping the patient develop trust in himself and in others. In implementing this phase of the strategy, the nurse may have to begin at "rock bottom" at the patient's primal need stage. That is, she may need to first help him meet his dependency needs, first the physiological ones and then the psychological, social and cultural ones. The nurse's reliability and credibility are demonstrated to the patient through nursing intervention. The interventions are directed toward alleviating problems arising from the simple, obvious activities of daily living or from the more complex, covert and unexpressed concerns of the individual. *The primary nursing care goal is to decrease feelings of insecurity and assist in establishing feelings of security.* Once the individual feels secure in the nurse-patient relationship, he can trust. The nurse fosters the growth of this initial trusting through specific planned actions. Three major nursing actions which promote trust are to show respect, to be honest and to provide consistency. Specific nursing activities which would exemplify these are included in Table 6-1.

TABLE 6-1
NURSING ACTIONS DESIGNED TO PROMOTE TRUST

Show Respect	Be Honest	Provide Consistency
1) Use the patient's proper name and title.	1) Keep promises.	1) Adhere to planned schedule.
2) Listen and give consideration to the patient's requests.	2) Be "open and above board" in words and actions.	2) Follow through on planned actions.

TABLE 6-1 (continued)

Show Respect	Be Honest	Provide Consistency
3) Allow for sufficient time to respond to questions.	3) Give reasons and explanations when requests cannot be met.	3) Adhere to set limitations.
4) Give clear instructions regarding procedures, policies and activities.	4) Consult with patients about their preferences.	4) Seek opportunities to pursue and foster the nurse-patient relationship outside of the regularly scheduled interaction session.
5) Openly acknowledge personal limitations in knowledge and ability.	5) Allow requests within limits of the situation.	
	6) Apologize for inconveniences.	
	7) Preserve confidentiality	

acknowledging and utilizing readiness

Readiness is also part of the process in the development of a relationship. It is an attitudinal and emotional state in which the individual is able to respond to the nurse. Readiness is based on the urgency to satisfy instinctual emotional needs. It is a demonstration of the patient's motivation to participate in the therapeutic process. There are several factors involved in the acknowledgment of the readiness. These include a statement of intention, an identification of the ultimate goal and a recognition of and appreciation for active participation in working toward the intended goal. The level of readiness depends upon the individual's degree of perception as well as his intellectual capacity. The exploitation aspect of readiness is significant because it is the foundation for the development of insight. Progression of the relationship is in direct proportion to the nurse's ability to take advantage of readiness and her ability to maximize opportunities to encourage and strengthen the relationship.

In determining readiness, the nurse must also consider the patient's level of anxiety since gross or uncontrolled anxiety inhibits the therapeutic alliance and problem solving. Nursing activity should be directed toward reducing anxiety to a manageable level. Some specific nursing actions which decrease anxiety are:

1 Planning and carrying out continuous contact with the patient over an extended period of time.
2 Listening attentively to the patient.
3 Keeping the nurse's responses to a minimum.
4 Responding clearly, briefly and specifically.

In some instances readiness may need to be encouraged by increasing the patient's anxiety by withdrawing support from the patient and thereby increasing his discomfort in an effort to motivate him to work on his problems. This is particularly true where the patient is highly dependent, procrastinates excessively or manipulates to avoid confronting problems or stresses. Specific nurse actions which increase the patient's anxiety level include:

1 Maintaining direct eye contact.

2 Delaying response to the patient's immediate need for gratification.

3 Ignoring superficial content by not responding.

4 Remaining silent when the patient is pressing for a personal opinion or decision from the nurse.

5 Introducing or focusing on topics that have been identified as emotionally charged.

6 Confronting the patient with an observation about his behavior.

Once the patient's readiness is identified by the nurse, there are certain nursing actions the nurse can employ to capitalize on this readiness and move with the patient to further develop the therapeutic relationship: she can be accessible, be concerned and provide comfort. Table 6-2 lists specific nursing activities to achieve these three actions.

TABLE 6-2
NURSING ACTIVITIES TO FACILITATE THE NURSE-PATIENT RELATIONSHIP

Be Accessible	Be Concerned	Provide Comfort
1) Approach at frequent intervals.	1) Display a willingness to become involved.	1) State the purpose of the relationship.
2) Designate specific times the nurse is available.	2) Display warmth and spontaneity.	2) Preserve confidentiality.
3) Allow for flexibility in schedule.	3) Encourage verbalizations.	3) State how shared material is to be used by self and other members of the health team.
4) Provide a private area where exploration of concerns can be pursued.	4) Encourage an expression of positive and negative feelings.	4) Clarify nursing role.
	5) Recognize verbal and nonverbal leads, clues or signals.	5) Give realistic and sincere responses.
	6) Focus on expressed concerns.	6) Allow patient to proceed at own rate.
		7) Follow through on stated goals.

setting limits

Setting limits is another strategy a nurse can use to permit exploration, growth and movement toward the development of the therapeutic nurse-patient relationship. *Setting limits* is the identification of boundaries both for the patient and for the nurse. It is the means by which the security of both patient and nurse are safeguarded. Setting limits is a structure which demonstrates its positive value through the reduction of anxiety. Setting limits provides a frame of reference that gives direction to choices and orientation for therapy. To be effective, setting limits must be a continuous process, consistently employed both on verbal and behavioral level.

The nurse must assume responsibility for clearly identifying limits in terms of time, person and place. Limits should be kept to a minimum and be consistent with the needs of the participants within the relationship. Specific nursing actions designed to implement the setting of limits are set out in Table 6-3.

TABLE 6-3
LIMIT SETTING

Time	Person	Place
1) Set specific appointment times.	1) Identify purposes and goals.	1) Select an appropriate place.
2) Be consistent in scheduling appointments.	2) Clarify the nursing role.	2) Be consistent with therapy location and atmosphere.
3) Start and end on time.	3) Keep the patient focused on therapy content and interaction.	3) Prevent interruptions.
4) Do not extend the session beyond the scheduled time.	4) Adhere to the specifics of the therapy contract.	

the nurse-patient relationship process

The nurse-patient relationship process is similar in structure to the communication process in that it is a planned series of events composed of steps which must be worked through and achieved before the next can be undertaken. The steps are orienting, working and terminating. Many references include another step termed "selection phase" which occurs prior to orientation. The rationale for including a selection phase is the belief that some patients can benefit therapeutically from a more intensive nurse-patient interaction than can others, thus requiring that the nurse make a decision with regard to who should and who should not receive therapy from her. We strongly feel, however, that *all* patients have a right to nursing care. The nurse-patient relationship is a therapeutic process involved in the delivery of nursing care, therefore, *all patients have a right and all nurses have an obligation* to engage in a therapeutic relationship with every patient. We advocate that nursing judgments not be in terms of selection of patients for a therapeutic relationship but rather be directed toward the selection of specific nurse-patient goals to be accomplished through this therapeutic relationship with each patient.

orienting

The nurse initiates the orientation period of the nurse-patient relationship. The purpose of this phase is to explore with the patient those concerns which seem to be most important to him. Although the nurse initiates the contact using a permissive approach, she also provides structure by identifying for the patient the purpose of the contact and by clarifying roles and expectations with regard to meeting place and length of time. Two major functions for the nurse during the orienting period are the observation and assessment of the patient and the creation of a therapeutic climate conducive to spontaneous verbalizations. These functions permit the nurse to collect data which will enable her to determine the patient's specific areas of difficulty in behavior and psychological functioning and thereby enable her to plan for effective nursing activity. The therapeutic tasks to be accomplished by the nurse in the orienting phase are to:

Foster a feeling of security through the continued building of trust.

Assist the patient to express verbally his thoughts and feelings.

Identify areas of inadequate functioning.

Assess areas of strengths and weaknesses.

Set priorities for nursing intervention.

working

The nurse-patient interaction enters the second step of the therapeutic relationship process when the patient is able to focus on the unpleasant and often painful aspects of his life. At this time, the patient demonstrates an ability to cope with the interpersonal demands of the therapeutic process. Together, the nurse and the patient concentrate on achieving the previously identified therapeutic goals. Nursing activity is directed toward increasing the normalcy of the patient's behavior. In other words, the nurse assists the patient to move toward his optimal level of functioning. The working phase is much more structured than the orienting phase. Now, the nurse assists the patient to focus on ideas, themes and emotional overtones, although structured, spontaneous interaction is encouraged. However, the nurse channels therapeutic communication toward the identified goals.

The therapeutic tasks to be accomplished by the nurse in the working phase are to:

Increase the individual's awareness and perception of the reality associated with his particular experiences.

Assist him in developing a realistic self-concept.

Promote his self-confidence.

Assist him in recognizing areas of discomfort and distress.

Increase his ability to verbally describe his feelings.

Assist him in his attempts to make comparisons.

Assist him in drawing conclusions regarding the comparisons.

Encourage him to select a realistic plan of action.

Provide opportunities for him to implement the plan of action.

Encourage him to evaluate the results of his behavior.

Assess his readiness.

Provide him with an opportunity for independent functioning.

terminating

The last phase of the nurse-patient relationship is the terminating phase. The therapeutic alliance is a singularly intimate and invested encounter. The patient tends to view the therapist as a powerful force in his life. Therefore, the nurse must be aware that when she engages in the process of termination with the patient, both of them need to work through and finalize this distinctly emotional and traumatic experience, which is generally referred to as separation anxiety. Termination is a gradual weaning process. It involves loss, separation, fear and anxiety. It often engenders feelings of discomfort, pain and anger and causes misplacement of feelings. Termination is initiated by mutual agreement when the patient demonstrates:

Ability to care for his personal physical needs and contribute to the maintenance of his environment.

Evidence of greater independence and ability to function without the nurse's support.

Increased ability to be self-governing.

Increased emotional stability over a period of time.

Increased self-esteem.

Ability to cope with frustration, anxiety and hostility.

The following situation typifies some of the problems and concerns of the patient when confronted with the reality of termination.

Mrs. Jones, a 43-year-old, Caucasian female came to a mental health clinic for complaints of general malaise and dissatisfaction with her job and her relationship with her second husband. Two children were born to the first marriage that ended in divorce seven years previous to her first Clinic appointment. A contract was made for Mrs. Jones to participate in twelve therapy sessions. After successful therapeutic engagement the contract was extended to include three termination sessions, one every two weeks. Mrs. Jones missed her second termination session. During the third scheduled appointment she began to complain bitterly about dissatisfaction and fear of others "ripping her off," as she had at the beginning of therapy. She stated that her work was not appreciated and neither would her teen-age daughter's work be appreciated in an approaching sewing contest. The nurse acknowledged Mrs. Jones' concerns and feelings and assisted her in ventilating negative feelings. Mrs. Jones requested a continuation of therapy. The nurse recognized the patient's feelings about termination. Mrs. Jones was obviously experiencing separation anxiety that, in turn, produced feelings of fear, anger, frustration and a sense of loss. These feelings were discussed with Mrs. Jones, who insisted that she needed more therapy. However, the therapist held to the original contract and therapy was terminated. Two weeks later Mrs. Jones called the nurse to announce that her daughter had won the sewing constest, her job was going so well that she was given a merit raise and that her marital relationship was "great."

The amount of time needed to accomplish the terminating phase is dependent on the duration of the relationship, the level of independent functioning achieved and the presence of unresolved problems. Generally, a nurse-patient relationship which has been in existence over a long period of time and which has been very intense requires a longer time span before termination can be achieved. Conversely, a brief, less intense relationship requires a shorter period of time. However, there are other factors which may tend to influence the rapidity with which termination takes place. Some of these factors include premature discharge, trial visit or transfer, the nurse's change in assignment, illness of either party, the nurse's vacation, or, in the case of a student, completion of a rotation. Even though these factors may tend to speed up the terminating phase, all the steps in the process itself must be followed in order for termination to be therapeutically effective. Since the primary task of the terminating process is dissolution of the relationship, the nurse must:

Space contracts with the patient further apart.

Decrease the amount of interaction time.

Establish a less intense, more relaxed atmosphere.

Focus on material that is future oriented.

Decline to respond to or follow up cues which could lead to new areas of exploration.

Provide for necessary referrals.

stumbling blocks and stepping stones

The student and beginning practitioner often encounter difficulties in implementing the processes involved in a therapeutic nurse-patient relationship. Many times the kinds of difficulties encountered arise out of the nurse's inexperience and anxiety. Major stumbling blocks frequently experienced occur in the areas of scheduling of appointments, methodology of recording, contract violations, hesitancy about dealing with feelings, over-realiance on stereotyped responses and inability to maintain the relationship on a therapeutic level. These trouble spots can be avoided or at least diminished in intensity and frequency. There are ways—stepping stones—by which the inexperienced practitioner can help herself to move more easily and comfortably into the therapeutic nurse-patient relationship. In Table 6-4 stumbling blocks expressed as "What if . . . ?" questions are answered by "Try this . . ." stepping stones.

TABLE 6-4
COMMON STUMBLING BLOCKS AND STEPPING STONES IN INITIATING AND MAINTAINING A THERAPEUTIC RELATIONSHIP

STUMBLING BLOCKS	STEPPING STONES
What if—	*Try this—*
1) the patient doesn't come to the session?	Locate the patient. Reschedule the appointment. Remind the patient ahead of time. Give the patient an appointment card.
2) the patient is habitually late?	Determine patient's orientation to time. Remind the patient of the approaching hour. Be on time and wait for the patient. Explore with the patient his reasons for lateness. Close the session on time.
3) the nurse is late or has to change the scheduled time?	Notify the patient directly or through another person or by a written message. Apologize. Reschedule when appropriate.
4) the patient asks to cut the session short or change the time of the meeting?	Explore the expressed need. Reorient the patient to the time schedule as per initial agreement. Reschedule when appropriate.
5) the patient abruptly leaves the session?	Ask, "Where are you going?" As the patient is leaving say, "I will wait until . . ." (the end of the session). Remain in the room. Wait expectantly for the patient's return—do not become involved in any other activity.

TABLE 6-4 (continued)

STUMBLING BLOCKS	STEPPING STONES
What if—	*Try this—*
6) the patient objects to the nurse's making notations?	Listen to the objections. Explain the purpose and use of note taking. Reinforce the positive concept of confidentiality. Matter of factly continue to record. Discontinue recording, write a summary immediately after the session.
7) the patient wants to read the notes?	Let him—he has the right.
8) the patient asks, "Who sees the notes?"	State clearly who will have access to the notes. Abide by the contract made with the patient.
9) other members of the staff ask to see the detailed notes?	Keep the staff informed as to the patient's progress. Refuse diplomatically to show detailed notes. Inform the staff of contract confidentiality.
10) the patient asks the nurse to give the notes to his doctor or other staff?	Explore with the patient the reasons for his request. Encourage the patient to speak for himself. Offer to accompany the patient and to support his interpersonal approaches with others.
11) the patient calls the nurse by her first name?	Recall to yourself the differences between a social and a therapeutic relationship. Not respond. Repeat your proper name and title. Explore reasons with patient. Reinforce the accepted policy used within the treatment setting.
12) the nurse wants to call the patient by his first name?	Review the differences between a social and a therapeutic relationship. Review the policy of the unit. Explore the request in light of the patient's ego identity.

TABLE 6-4 (continued)

STUMBLING BLOCKS	STEPPING STONES
What if—	*Try this—*
13) the patient asks personal questions?	Briefly answer factual and self-evident questions. Explore with the patient his need to ask. Redirect the focus of communication toward patient.
14) the sessions are interrupted by patients or staff?	Clearly state to interrupting individual that a therapy session is in progress. Place a "Do Not Disturb" or "Therapy in Session" sign on the door.
15) the patient doesn't want to talk?	Sit quietly. Look at patient with an interested, expectant expression. Observe nonverbal behavior. Use indirect, open-ended statements at intervals, such as, "You seem to be thinking . . ." Remind the patient of the remaining time: "You still have fifteen minutes."
16) the patient says, "I have nothing to say," or "I don't know"?	Rephrase the question. Learn to sit quietly and wait and be patient. Recognize and deal with your own feelings evoked by the patient's response. Remain optimistic. Continue to explore areas of interest and concern. Be persistent—don't give up.
17) the nurse uses the same responses over and over again?	Vary responses. Deal with resultant rejection. Deal with patient's anger. Deal with patient's avoidance of you. Review and analyze your notes: —look for stereotyped nurse responses. —look for missed cues. —rephrase nurse responses. —try out alternatives in next session. Be sensitive to mistakes and learn from them. Consult with instructor, head nurse or member of the interdisciplinary team.

TABLE 6-4 (continued)

STUMBLING BLOCKS	STEPPING STONES
What if—	*Try this—*
18) the patient tells the nurse to go away or says, "Don't bother me!"	Remain calm. Assess the patient's level of hostility. Make judgments based on the assessment and act accordingly: —leave patient with a promise to return at a later time, or —remain and explore patient's feelings.
19) the nurse's questions upset the patient or make him more "nervous"?	Good—something's happening. Maintain focus on the topic—don't avoid it: —identify the topic. —help patient to recognize the topic to the patient's therapeutic advantage. Review and analyze data to prevent: —prying. —pushing beyond the patient's level of readiness.

suggested readings

Arnold, Helen M. "Working With Schizophrenic Patients." *American Journal of Nursing,* Vol. 76 No. 6 (June, 1976), 941-943.

Benjamin, Alfred. *The Helping Interview.* Houghton Mifflin Co.: Boston, 1969.

Bermosk, Loretta Sue, and Mordan, Mary Jane. *Interviewing in Nursing.* MacMillan Co.: New York, 1964.

Bernstein, Lewis, and Dana, Richard H. *Interviewing and the Health Professions.* Appleton-Century Crofts: New York, 1970.

Bochnak, Mary, et al. "The Comparison of Two Types of Nursing Activity in the Relief of Pain." *Innovations in Nurse-Patient Relationships: Automatic or Reasoned Nurse Actions.* American Nurses Association: New York, 1962, 5-11.

Burkett, Alice D. "A Way to Communicate." *American Journal of Nursing,* Vol. 73 No. 12 (December, 1973), 2185-2187.

Cameron, Joyce. "The Patient Needs to Be Understood." *Nursing and The Patient's Motivations.* American Nursing Association: New York, 1962, 5-13.

Colbert, Lucy. "Debra Finds Herself." *Nursing Outlook,* Vol. 19 No. 1 (January, 1971), 50-52.

Dillon, Kathryn. "A Patient—Structured Relationship." *Perspectives in Psychiatric Care,* Vol. 9 No. 4 (1971), 167-172.

Gahan, Karen A. "Problem Solving as a Therapeutic Process." *Journal of Psychiatric Nursing and Mental Health Services,* Vol. 14 No. 11 (November, 1976), 37-39.

Kopacz, Marcia Socksteder and O'Connor, Sister Catherine M. "Through A Glass Darkly". *American Journal of Nursing,* Vol. 75 No. 12 (December, 1975), 2159-2160.

Lewis, Garland K. *Nurse–Patient Communications.* Wm. C. Brown: Debuque, Iowa, 1969.

Meldman, Newman, Schaller, and Peterson. "Patients' Responses to Nurse-Psychotherapists." *American Journal of Nursing,* Vol. 71 No. 6 (June 1971) 1150-51.

Mellow, June. "Nursing Therapy." *American Journal of Nursing,* Vol. 68 No. 11 (November, 1968) 2365.

Mercer, Lianne S., and O'Connor, Patricia. *Fundamental Skills in the Nurse-Patient Relationship.* W. B. Saunder Co.: Philadelphia, 1969.

Mooney, Judith. "Attachment/Separation in the Nurse-Patient Relationship." *Nursing Forum,* Vol. 15 No. 3 (1976), 2959-2964.

O'Brien, Maureen J. *Communications and Relationships.* C. V. Mosbey Co.: St. Louis, 1974.

Orlando, Ida Jean. *The Dynamic Nurse-Patient Relationship.* G. P. Putnam's Sons: New York, 1961.

Rogers, Carl. *On Becoming a Person.* Houghton Mifflin Co.: Boston, 1961.

Rogers, Carl. *Client-Centered Therapy.* Houghton Mifflin Co.: Boston, 1951.

Shertzer, Bruce, and Stone, Shelley C. *Fundamentals of Counseling.* Houghton Mifflin Co.: Boston, 1968.

Simmons, Janet A. *The Nurse-Client Relationship in Mental Health Nursing.* W. B. Saunders Co.: Philadelphia, 1976.

Soupe, Paul. "How Do You Feel Nurse?" *American Journal of Nursing,* Vol. 74 No. 6 (June, 1974), 1105.

Travelbee, Joyce. *Interpersonal Aspects of Nursing.* F. A. Davis Co.: Philadelphia, 1966.

———. *Intervention in Psychiatric Nursing.* F. A. Davis Co.: Philadelphia, 1970.

Uhjely, Gertrud B. *Determinants of the Nurse–Patient Relationship.* Springer Publishing Co., Inc.: New York, 1968.

———. "Two Types of Problem Patients and How to Deal with Them." *Nursing 76,* Vol. 6 No. 5 (May, 1976), 64-67.

chapter 7

groups: their purpose, structure and operation

learning objectives

On completion of this chapter the reader should be able to:

1 Define the term *group*.
2 Realize the importance that groups play in the life of an individual.
3 Understand the benefits of group experience.
4 Identify distinguishing features of group structure.

purpose and importance

A *group* is a unit of society composed of two or more people in interaction. Groups are formed to meet the social, emotional and physical needs of individuals. The individual achieves healthy development through appropriate group life experiences throughout his entire life. Just as an individual learns about individual interpersonal relationships from his "significant other," so he learns his interpersonal group relationships from the initial primary group, his family. His family's interaction with him and with others, as a unit of society, serves as a model on which he bases other group interactions. In fact, the individual's successful development of his own satisfying life style depends on his ability to relate well with others. Groups have power to support individual effort and accomplishment; reject behavior which does not conform to group values, norms or expectations; foster creativity and deal with critical issues which impede individual or group progress. Groups provide the mechanism for the resolution of interpersonal conflicts in all levels of human interaction.

When an individual moves into a group experience he expands the facets of his own personality. His uniqueness as an individual is enhanced by the collective presence of all other members of the group. As an individual operates within a group situation, he identifies with others, and this bond provides a reciprocal influence between the self and the group. The group is never merely a sum of its individual members or parts, but takes on an added dimension that is a composite of the diversities of the group members. But a group is more than a composite of various personalities; the reciprocal influence each member exerts on the others causes individuals to assimilate the characteristics of the group.

In Chapter Four, interpersonal relationships were identified in terms of group types: primary, secondary and tertiary. A *group* is a joint enterprise in which mutual need gratification and interdependency exists between and among group members. Simultaneously, an individual usually belongs to at least one primary group and to one or more secondary and tertiary groups. These secondary and tertiary interpersonal group relationships are commonly referred to as reference-group relationships.

A child begins his group experience with birth when he joins his parents and siblings. Together they form a primary group. During infancy and the preschool period, the family, as the initial primary group, sets the stage for the child's future group experiences. When the child begins school his classmates and teachers make up another potential primary interpersonal group. With the broadening of the child's living experiences through introduction of new or expanded group participation there is a proportionate increase in the range and selectivity of his relationships. There is also a visible increase in his emotional and intellectual growth. Thus, group experiences have a two-fold effect in the early stages of life. First, as the child develops relationships within the group, the child develops distinction as a person; and second, as the child participates in group interaction, he is in turn stimulated to explore his environment and grow further.

With pre-adolescence and adolescence, group participation becomes closely aligned with the physical process of maturation and the psychological quest for independence. At this stage of development, the allegiances, mores, attitudes and behavioral patterns of the peer group tend to surpass and surplant family and school as the primary learning group. Peer-group involvement is an important aspect in the growth and developmental scheme of an individual's personality in that it facilitates social growth and value system integration, which in turn leads to participation in the broader spectrum of adult society.

Primary and reference groups are ever present and changing throughout the individual's life. Group experiences are essential to the psycho-social development of the individual. Participation in groups facilitates the maturation of relationships between the individual and society. These relationships are analagous to mechanisms the individual can use to assist in the attainment of self-actualization.

If, as stated above, group experiences are essential, how do they contribute to the development of a healthy, functioning member of society? Group experiences are beneficial in that they provide the individual with the following:

> A basis for identification with peers.
>
> A means by which the interpersonal needs for acceptance, recognition and control can be met.
>
> The freedom "to be," that is, the ability to express self without fear of censure or retaliation, along with the freedom to be different in the presence of others.
>
> The freedom to choose and form a deeper and more intimate relationship with individuals within the group.

In addition, group experiences permit and provide the individual with opportunities to:

> Exercise independence while remaining secure in the knowledge that dependency needs will also be met.
>
> Develop interpersonal skills as a participating member of society.
>
> Evaluate skills with respect to the individual's ability to learn and to achieve.
>
> Formulate attitudes and values.
>
> Set goals for self.
>
> Experiment.

structure

The composition of any group depends on the purpose of the group. Groups are composed of people who have vested interests, common concerns, and mutual needs. Groups form, merge, disintegrate and reorganize based on gratification of needs and realization of goals. Ideally, group composition reflects a membership sufficiently similar enough to provide the participants with mutual support yet different enough to expose the participants to stimulation and motivation for continued active membership.

Although group composition may vary according to size, types of membership and purpose, there are certain features of group membership and behavior that remain constant and contribute to the success of groups. These features include the individuals' status within the group; the roles chosen by the individuals or designated by the group; the norms and values exhibited by the group; and the kind of flexibility, communication patterns and cohesiveness maintained.

status

Status is the prestige of an individual member within a group in relationship to other members. Status designates prominence within the group in relationship to all other members and is bestowed on the individual by consensus of the group. It designates a person's position, influences his degree of effectiveness in carrying out his role and increases the power the individual is able to exert. Status is arbitrary and subject to change. Fluctuation in status is often governed by the addition or subtraction of group members, modification of group goals or changes in members' roles.

role and role function

Role is the "part" an individual plays in group life. A role may be assigned or assumed. An assigned role is one which is delegated by the group to satisfy a group need, whereas the assumed role is taken on by the individual member to satisfy his needs. Role depends on the expectations the individual brings to the group with respect to self and the expectations for the relationship the self has with others. To accomplish a specific group task, roles may sometimes be exchanged among members. Role functions are those operations or activities which exemplify a given role.

Specific roles which may be found in any given group situation would most likely include the following.

leader

The *leader* is a coordinator. Leadership encompasses three facets— managerial ability, technical adroitness, and expertise in human relations. The leader is that individual group member who demonstrates ability in organizing and making use of the capabilities of group members to achieve the specific tasks or goals of the group. A successful leader is able to accept and follow through on the responsibility for group performance. The leader must also demonstrate an ability to hold group members accountable for their specific tasks within the group. Other traits displayed by a successful group leader include self-directiveness, initiative, dependability, conscientiousness, adaptability and sensitivity to group climate. Group leadership requires the ability to perform any and all functions which enables the group to achieve its goal, promotes group viability, maintains and encourages people-to-people interaction and increases interdependence among group members. Leadership may be acquired in one of two ways, either by formal appointment or through the natural selection of an emerging group.

Some specific role functions which are required of a leader are:

Initiating action.
Clarifying issues.
Focusing on goals.

Supplying data necessary to facilitate group function.

Mediating issues.

Assisting in defining member roles and functions.

Evaluating group member performance.

Providing for encouragement and recognition of group members.

Allowing and encouraging active participation by all members, especially those that hold minority viewpoints.

Promoting effective patterns of communication.

Providing for a mechanism for accurate report keeping.

Encouraging mutual trust, respect and warmth.

follower

The *follower* is a group member who fulfills a specific role and performs role functions in relationship to the type of group, its purpose and goals. Each group member contributes uniquely to the group. There are many different sub roles within a given group that members can assume; however, not all of these roles are present in every group. Some of the more common roles which occur consistently in groups are listed below.

Diplomat—the member who makes himself responsible for maintaining group harmony. The diplomat displays a high degree of sensitivity regarding the individual needs of group members. He employs tact in the resolution of potential discord and attempts to reconcile disagreements.

Humorist—the member who makes himself responsible for releasing group tension. The humorist effectively applies exaggeration and satire to provide comic relief which results in the dissipation of mounting anxiety, frustration or hostility.

Liaison—the member who makes himself responsible for communicating the needs, concerns and issues of the group between the group and outside authorities. He is a spokesman for the group who relays clear and concise messages to and from the group.

Specialist—the member who makes himself responsible for meeting the particular requirements of the group. The specialist acts as a resource person who provides information and access to such things as activities, commodities, donations or funds.

Listener—the group member who makes himself responsible for "lending an ear" and acting as confidant to troubled group members. The listener demonstrates friendliness, warmth and sympathy. The listener is highly responsive to the individual needs of group members.

Talker—the group member who feels responsible for maintaining communication in the group. He makes use of every opportunity to expound on all issues and has a tendency to be repetitive. This behavior can generate agitation and negative feelings toward the talker. If left unchecked it can produce disintegration and/or goal failure within the group. In other instances the talker through his incessance allows other group members to daydream or lose sight of group goals.

Silent participant—the group member who assumes an inconspicuous place within the group. The silent participant hesitates to draw attention to himself; however, when called upon, contributes to the total functioning of the group.

norms and values

Group norms are rules governing the actions of group members. They are established within the group, for the group and are enforced by group consensus. Group norms spell out the criteria for the procedural activity of the group, such as how decisions are to be made and implemented and which member will fulfill what role. A *group value* is the shared belief of the group. Values held by the group are consciously operational and have both a moral and motivating aspect. The moral aspect enables the group to collectively assess the appropriateness or inappropriateness of either individual action within the group or the joint action of the whole group. This moral aspect offers guidelines and encouragement for specific behaviors or postures to be carried out or assumed by the group in its operations. Group values, although collectively operational for the group, may vary for a particular individual within the group. Differences in values among individual group members are generally acceptable to the group; however, differences in norms among individual members of the group are generally not acceptable to the group.

flexibility

Group flexibility is the ability the group possesses to adapt and grow as a collective body. The degree of flexibility within any given group is based on the degree of understanding that each individual member has for all other members of the group. As a group which is flexible encounters new experiences, new problems, or sees new dimensions to its stated goals or purpose it can mobilize the specialized capabilities of its individual members in accomplishing the group goal. In a flexible group, each member knows when to take the initiative and when to follow.

communication patterns

Group communication patterns are those channels through which individual members of the group rely and receive information pertinent to the collective functioning of the group. The communication pattern within a group is the mechanism for interpersonal interaction, that is, the way *who* says *what* to *whom* and *when*. The communication pattern must allow for openness and honesty. An effective communication pattern provides the individual member with a feeling of security—security in the knowledge that when he sets forth his ideas and feelings and exposes his inner self to collective group inspection he will not experience rejection, retaliation or invalidation.

cohesiveness

Group cohesiveness is the demonstration of attraction that members have for each other in terms of kinship. It is the group working together as a collective unit and an expression of the desire to remain together as a unified whole. Group cohesion contributes to the viability and efficacy of the group. It increases the interpersonal rewards for individual members of the group by supplying gratification for recognition, approval and support. Group cohesion promotes group mobility toward fulfilling group goals.

suggested readings

Berne, Eric. *Games People Play*. Ballantine Books, Inc.: New York, 1964.

Cartwright, Darwin, and Zander, Alvin. *Group Dynamics*. Harper & Row Publishers: New York, 1968.

Gardner, Kathryn. "Patient Groups in a Therapeutic Community." *American Journal of Nursing*, Vol. 71 No. 3 (March, 1971), 528-532.

Hare, Paul, Borgatte, Edgar F., and Balec, Robert F. *Small Groups—Studies in Social Interaction*. Alfred A. Knopf: New York, 1962.

Hendrik, M. Reutenbeck. *The New Group Therapies*. Avon Book Company: New York, 1970.

Homans, George C. *The Human Group*. Harcourt, Brace & Co.: New York, 1950.

Kempf, Florence C., and Useem, Ruth Hill. *Psychology Dynamics of Behavior in Nursing*. W. B. Saunders Co.: Philadelphia, 1964.

Merton, Robert K. "The Social Nature of Leadership," *American Journal of Nursing* (December, 1969), 2614-2618.

Racy, John. "How A Group Grows." *American Journal of Nursing*, Vol. 69 No. 11 (November, 1969), 2396-2402.

Rogers, Carl. *Client-Centered Therapy—Its Current Practice, Implications and Theory*. Houghton Mifflin Co.: Boston, 1951.

Roucek, Joseph S., and Warren, L. Roland. *Sociology Introductions*. Littlefield Adams & Co.: Ames, Iowa, 1953.

Ruesch, Jurgen, and Bateson, Gregory. *Communication: The Social Matrix of Psychiatry*. W. W. Norton & Co., Inc.: New York, 1968.

Shepherd, Clovis R. *Small Groups: Some Sociological Perspectives*. Chandler Publishing Co.: Scranton, Pa., 1964.

Slavson, S. R. *Introduction to Group Therapy*. International Universities Press Inc.: New York, 1965.

Theelen, Herbert A. *Dynamics of Groups at Work*. University of Chicago Press: Chicago, 1954.

chapter 8

group process

learning objectives

On completion of this chapter the reader should be able to:

1 Understand the definition, process and dynamics of group therapy.
2 Become acquainted with the types of therapeutic groups.
3 Identify the nurse's role and responsibility for initiating and conducting therapeutic groups.
4 Recognize impediments to the therapeutic group process.
5 Implement specific intervention for the success of the therapeutic group process.

definition and purpose

Group therapy is a structured or semistructured process of therapeutic intervention in which the behavioral and emotional reactions of the individual members of the group, toward each other and toward the leader, are acknowledged and understood as projections of individual interpersonal distress. Participation in group therapy provides a re-educational experience, in which the individual as a "separate self" and the group as a "collective self" are involved in a process of learning and problem solving for the purpose of dealing with the emotional and behavioral reactions necessary to the production of change within themselves and with the group.

There are significant differences between a social group and a therapeutic group. These differences occur in four major areas—organization, membership, composition and use of the leadership role—shown in Table 8-1.

TABLE 8-1
MAJOR DISTINGUISHING CHARACTERISTICS BETWEEN
SOCIAL AND THERAPEUTIC GROUPS

Social Group	Therapeutic Group
Organization	
Casual, most often for diversional, professional or religious activities.	Purposeful, educative, interventive and preventative.
For a variety of reasons dependent on needs or interests.	Specific change objective in mind.
Membership	
Varies in terms of numbers, purpose or goals.	Limited to persons experiencing some difficulty in coping with emotional stress.
	Limited to those seeking therapeutic assistance.
Composition	
More likely to have a heterogeneous mixture.	Occasionally heterogeneous.
More likely to be representative of a cross section of society.	Deliberate selection is based on specific factors such as age, sex, marital status, presenting problem, and specific needs.
Leadership Role	
Usually by election, appointment, or consensus.	Therapist is the primary group leader.
Less well-defined.	Clearly structured and defined.
Flexible.	Employs specific therapeutic leadership tasks.
	Implements and guides therapeutic process.
	Emphasizes therapeutic process over the social process.

process

Group effectiveness is a direct result of the educational process that exists and develops between the therapist (group leader) and the group members.

However, the therapist's involvement in the process is not a guarantee of success in and of itself. The therapist must cultivate certain factors in the group process that encourage and enhance change. These factors include:

1 *Sharing information*—the mutual exchange of relevant data which provides a basis for understanding.

2 *Hope*—the belief in self and in the process that help and comfort is available, that at the end of the tunnel there is the light of acceptance, understanding, relief and recovery.

3 *Universality*—security in the knowledge that "my problem," feelings and behaviors are known, felt and shared by others. It is the idea that the self is not alone in its distress, not "so different."

4 *Altruism*—an unselfish interest in others and their well-being. It is the expression of mutual concern, support, recognition, comfort, assurance and respect among the members of the group.

5 *Transference of primary group images and relationships*—the therapeutic group is substituted for the initial primary group and may be compared to the initial primary group, the family. This comparison and substitution permits the individual to nullify past learned group interaction and expectations and create for himself a new set of experiences and expectations.

6 *Socialization*—a process in which the techniques and skills necessary for social interaction are explored, experimented with and evaluated within the context of the group, by the group. The outcome of socialization is learning new patterns of acceptable social interaction.

7 *Ventilation*—an active verbal participation in the group process through the use of self-disclosure and self-exploration. It provides the individual member with an opportunity to test his concepts, validate his ideas and feelings, and re-evaluate them in light of the responses obtained from his fellow group members.

group dynamics

Group therapy differs from individual therapy in that group therapy more closely approximates a broader cross section of social or emotional experiences. In addition, group therapy makes use of comprehensive social interaction. These two factors give group therapy the added benefit of providing feedback that is derived from a multiplicity of responses. Regardless of the types of group, specialized needs or therapeutic goals, there is a mechanism of operation which consistently occurs. This mechanism is divided into four stages: the stage of group formation and organization; the stage of group cohesion; the stage of group interaction; and the stage of group dissolution.

the stage of group formation and organization

This stage is that period of time in which the therapist scrutinizes the patient population in reference to patient needs and problems that can best be served through the group process. Consideration is given to homogeneity of needs and problems; age and sex of participants; goals to be achieved; contract of time; the patient's ability and willingness to participate in the group process; and the optimal number of participants. Manageable and optimal group numbers should, theoretically, never exceed ten.

the stage of group cohesion

This stage covers that period of time it takes group members to become acquainted. During this period of testing the members behave as strangers and are cautiously polite to each other. During this time there is discussion of who the members are, their reasons for being in the group and identification of possible goals. This stage is characterized by conflict and lack of unity. The members demonstrate distrust and covert hostility. These projected feelings are directed toward individual members as well as toward the therapist. When the membership begins to interact more openly and positively with one another, the group, together with the leader, moves into the second stage.

the stage of group interaction

Hostility and anxiety become more overt in this stage. Feelings and expressed concerns are dealt with more directly by the group. As similarities are identified and discussed, thoughts and feelings revealed, and conflicts and frustrations handled, group cohesiveness develops. As group cohesiveness increases there is a proportionate increase in the productivity of the group. The result of increased group cohesiveness and productivity is a change in the communication pattern. No longer do individual group members speak directly to individuals; they now address themselves to the entire group. This intergroup communication pattern enhances the opportunity for emotional and social re-education. The group is able to focus its attention on fulfilling the identified therapeutic goals.

the stage of group dissolution

This stage begins as the therapeutic tasks of the group near completion. It is that period of time necessary to bring about effective dissolution of group relationships. During this stage group members face and cope with the feelings associated with loss and separation anxiety. Members freely express feelings of being abandoned, rejected or forsaken. Effective resolution depends on the group's ability to cope with these painful expressions. Because of the developed emotional maturity of the group which results from the second stage of the group, it is now able to be mutually supportive during this crisis period and successfully complete the final therapeutic task of closure.

types of therapy groups:

Within the scope of group therapy three points of reference can be distinguished which serve as a basis for determining the type of group therapy most effective to meet particular needs. These points of reference include:

1 The theroetical framework under which the group operates.
2 The particular characteristics or nature of the group members.
3 The therapeutic task to be accomplished.

Generally, throughout the literature reference is made to various modalities of the therapeutic group intervention. Table 8-2 is a synthesis and comparison of what we perceive to be the major types.

the nurse's role in group therapy

There are many different kinds of approaches that can be utilized in the practice of group therapy and many different types of group therapies. Each method is distinctive and has its own particular characteristics and expected sets of outcomes. Nonetheless, whatever approach the nurse group therapist chooses, there are specific nurse-leader behaviors which are fundamental and universal. These behaviors may be viewed in terms of attitudes, abilities and functions or tasks.

attitudes

The type of attitude the nurse therapist needs to cultivate is one which expresses to the group realistic, hopeful, therapeutic expectations for success and change. The nurse conveys to the group, through this attitude, her commitment and concern. The nurse reacts with thoughtfulness, simplicity and honesty, demonstrating by her actions a willingness to share in the responsibilities of the group work. The nurse therapist's attitude toward the group should clearly indicate that every person within the group, without exception, is the most important person there. Whatever the individual says or does not say is significant within the context of the experiences of the group.

abilities

The nurse group therapist must possess skills and abilities needed by leaders of any kind of group. In addition, the nurse therapist needs therapeutic skills. These would include the skillful use of therapeutic communication

TABLE 8-2
TYPES OF THERAPY GROUPS

	Didactic—Inspirational	Interventive—Exploratory	Activity
Definition	A group process which places emphasis on an educational experience designed to foster intellectual and emotional exchange while reflecting ethical, religious or societal values	A group process which encourages group members to verbally express and examine emotional or psychological problems within the context of their past and present individual and group interpersonal relationships.	A group process which emphasizes social interaction versus verbal interaction among group members and which encourages the development of ego strengths and control.
Goal	Better adaptation to environment through education and inspiration.	Development of insight leading to adaptation, modification or reconstruction of personality structure and/or behavior patterns.	Development of the socialization process; better adaptation to physical and social environment; and opportunity to test out relationships within a non-threatening environment.
Theoretical Base	Learning theory; Behavior modification; Biofeedback	Analytic theory Neo-Freudian theory Behavioral theory Gestalt psychology Reality therapy Transactional analysis	Social theory behavior Modification milieu therapy Nonverbal communication theory
Primary Therapeutic Role Function	Provide information Encourage discussion Support existing coping mechanism and defenses Persuade members to solve a specific type of problem Promote group solidarity and comradeship	Encourage the expression of ideas and the ventilation of feelings Confront existing defenses Assist in the development or modification of coping mechanisms Offer reassurance, empathy and feedback to group members.	Plan, organize and coordinate social, recreational, occupational and industries activities Identify and reinforce previous interests Promote the development of new outlets

TABLE 8-2 (continued)

	Didactic—Inspirational	Interventive—Exploratory	Activity
Examples	1) Discharge planning group 2) Recovery, Incorporated 3) Alcoholics Anonymous 4) Sex education 5) Health education 6) Rap group 7) Synanon 8) Prenatal instructional group 9) Ostomy Club 10) Dietary instruction group	1) T Group 2) Encounter group 3) Psychodrama 4) Family therapy 5) Intensive psychotherapy 6) Marital counseling 7) Adolescent therapy 8) Adjustment to disability of handicaps group	1) Current events group 2) Remotivational group 3) Reality orientation 4) Music therapy 5) Play therapy 6) Art therapy 7) Body building or exercise group 8) Excursion group

process; technical expertise in the maintenance and promotion of group interaction; an awareness of the dynamics of group process; the ability to interpret and integrate behavior within the context of group experiences; and the ability to intervene on behalf of individual members. Other abilities necessary for successful nurse therapist leadership include an awareness of self and the part self plays in the context of group interaction; recognition and resolution of the nurse-therapist's own internal conflicts; and, last but not least, the capacity for empathy.

The nurse-therapist leadership role in group therapy involves having role functions as a group member, but maintaining a distinct line between the patient and nonpatient role. In any initial group therapy contact, the nurse-therapist is automatically identified and looked to as "leader"; however, it is the skill and ability the nurse therapist exercises which enables her to maintain the leadership role and, through it, maintain the control or direction of the group toward its therapeutic purpose goal.

functions or tasks

We have identified five major functions with their associated tasks. They are as follows.

- I Formation of the group
    1 Select potential participants based on predetermined criteria.
    2 Conduct an interview with each potential participant.
    3 Present to potential participants the selected purpose and goals of the group.
    4 Assess ability of potential participants to meet criteria and their willingness to participate.
    5 Finalize selection of group members.
- II Organization of the group
    1 Select appropriate time and place.
    2 Arrange for record keeping.
    3 Encourage members to attend.
    4 Convene the group.
    5 Introduce group members.
    6 Restate and clarify purpose and goals.
    7 Identify limits.
    8 Initiate the development of group norms and values.
    9 Encourage spontaneous participation.
- III Recognition of themes of individual sessions
    1 Listen skillfully.
    2 Be actively involved in the developing group process.

    3 Clarify verbal and nonverbal communication.

    4 Invest, explore, validate and evaluate content

IV Development of common shared perceptions

    1 Identify individual perceptions.

    2 Investigate and explore possible similarities and differences.

    3 Encourage and support group interface.

    4 Assist and support group members in their search for group consensus.

V Assessment of physical and motor activity

    1 Recognize and identify any increase in the level of verbal and nonverbal activity.

    2 Identify and analyze possible and probable causes.

    3 Validate interpretations with the group.

    4 Intervene to exercise control either by supporting an individual member or by limit setting.

stumbling blocks and stepping stones

Just as the nurse practitioner has difficulty in initiating her role as therapist with patients on a one-to-one basis, so too the beginning nurse group leader also encounters some therapeutic difficulties in the implementation of an actual group session. Some of the common stumbling blocks the nurse group leader is likely to encounter along with some stepping stones that will assist in enabling her to deal with these difficulties are presented in Table 8-3.

TABLE 8-3
COMMON STUMBLING BLOCKS AND STEPPING STONES ASSOCIATED WITH GROUP THERAPY

STUMBLING BLOCKS	STEPPING STONES
What if—	*Try this—*
1) the prospective group members demonstrate initial resistance to attending the group?	Encourage patient to verbalize his negative feelings. Listen intently. Accept expressed thoughts and feelings without judgment or criticism. Restate and clarify purpose. Suggest that the patient "give it a try."
2) all members of group try to talk at once?	Stop the interaction and regain control of group by stating, "Everyone is talking at once."

TABLE 8-3 (continued)

STUMBLING BLOCKS	STEPPING STONES
What if—	*Try this—*
	Explore with the group possible causes for behavior.
	Encourage recognition of individual speakers.
	Focus therapist's attention on individuals when they speak.
	Review and re-establish the "ground rules."
3) one person monopolizes the discussion?	Allow the group to intervene and set limits if they are able.
	Interrupt positively and request another group member to give his opinion about what is being said.
	Explore the feelings of the group when one member talks all the time.
4) a group member uses excessive profanity, causing disruption?	Exercise control and impose limits.
	Enforce the limits.
5) the patients are negative to limit setting?	Remain firm—don't back down.
	Request the patient to leave the group until he regains self-control.
	Set up an individual session to explore the patient's feelings.
	Encourage the individual to maintain group membership.
6) a group member is verbally aggressive toward the therapist?	Set an example by maintaining your "cool."
	Absorb hostility.
	Speak in a low, even tone.
	Maintain eye contact if possible.
	Identify the angry feeling.
	Assist the patient to recognize his anger.
7) a group member is verbally aggressive toward another member?	Sit still and observe—avoid taking sides.
	Allow time for group members to exert control.
	Determine group feeling about the aggressiveness.
	Distract attention by focusing on feeling.
	Act as arbitrator.
	Deflect hostility by acting as a buffer between aggressor and group.
8) the group is not progressing?	Re-evaluate data with a colleague consultant.

TABLE 8-3 (continued)

STUMBLING BLOCKS	STEPPING STONES
What if—	*Try this—*
	Review with the group progress to date with respect to initial framework.
	Explore with the group reasons for lack of productivity.
	Re-affirm group objectives and goals.
	Ask for suggestions from the group for reaching the goals.
9) a task-oriented group cannot reach a consensus?	Summarize positions or data already presented.
	Keep focus on immediate concern.
	Encourage the group to explore alternatives.
10) a member of the group is rejected by the group?	Focus attention of group away from "rejected member."
	Demonstrate therapist acceptance by supporting group member's attempt to become part of the group.
	Give recognition to isolated member when merited.
	Assist the group to identify cause for group behavior toward rejected member.
	Re-evaluate the isolated member's readiness for group participation.
	Consider these possible alternatives:
	—remove the individual from the group.
	—transfer him to another group.
	—set up individual therapy.
	—confront group with the group's behavior toward the isolated member.
11) a member negatively manipulates?	Ignore the manipulative behavior.
	Treat the disruptive behavior matter of factly.
	Restate positively expectations in relationship to group goals.
12) a member discloses highly emotionally charged data about himself?	Elicit feelings of group members about the data.
	Identify any changes in the membership's attitude or opinions toward the sharing person.
	Maintain the therapeutic objective self toward the sharing member.
	Remind membership that they are bound by confidentiality outside the group.

suggested readings

Armacost, Betty, et al. "A Group of Problem Patients." *American Journal of Nursing*, Vol. 74 No. 2 (February, 1974), 289-292.

Armstrong, Shirley W., and Rouslin, Sheila. *Group Psychotherapy in Nursing Practice*. The Macmillan Co.: New York, 1963.

Authier, Jerry, and Gustafson, Kay. "Group Intervention Techniques: A Practical Guide for Psychiatric Team Members." Journal of Psychiatric and Mental Health Services, Vol. 14 No. 7 (July, 1976), 19-22.

Babcock, Dorothy E. "Transactional Analysis." *American Journal of Nursing*, Vol. 76 No. 7 (July, 1976), 1152-1155.

Brooks, Dorothy D. "Teletherapy: or How to Use Videotape Feedback to Enhance Group Process." *Perspectives in Psychiatric Care*, Vol. 14 No. 2 (1976), 83-87.

Burgess, Ann Wolbert, and Lazare, Aaron. *Psychiatric Nursing in the Hospital and the Community*. Prentice-Hall, Inc.: Englewood Cliffs, New Jersey, 1976.

Conte, Andrea, et al. "Group Work With Hypertensive Patients." *American Journal of Nursing*, Vol. 74 No. 5 (May, 1974), 910-912.

Friedman, Alfred M., and Kaplan, Harold I. eds. *Comprehensive Textbook of Psychiatry*. The Williams & Wilkins Co.: Baltimore, 1967.

Fochtman, Grace. "Therapeutic Factors of the Informal Group." *American Journal of Nursing*, Vol. 76 No. 2 (February, 1976), 238-239.

Goldberg, Connie, and Stanitis, Mary Anne. "The Enhancement of Self-Esteem Through the Communication Process in Group Therapy." *The Journal of Psychiatric Nursing and Mental Health Seminar*, Vol. 5 No. 12 (December, 1977), 5-8.

Johnson, James A. *Group Therapy A Practical Approach*. McGraw-Hill Book Co., Inc.: New York, 1963.

Kempf, Florence C., and Useem, Ruth Hill. *Psychology Dynamics of Behavior in Nursing*. W. B. Saunders Co.: Philadelphia, 1964.

Lancaster, Jeanette. "Activity Groups as Therapy." *American Journal of Nursing*, Vol. 76 No. 6 (June, 1976), 947-949.

Lyon, Glu Gamble. "Stimulation Through Motivation." *American Journal of Nursing*, Vol. 71 No. 5 (May, 1971), 982-985.

Morgan, Arthur James, and Moreno, Judith Wilson. *The Practice of Mental Health Nursing: A Community Approach*. J. B. Lippincott Co.: Philadelphia, 1973.

Parsell, Sue, and Lagliareni, Elaine Mary. "Cancer Patients Help Each Other." *American Journal of Nursing*, Vol. 74 No. 4 (April, 1974), 650-651.

Robinson, Lisa. *Psychiatric Nursing as a Human Experience*. W. B. Saunders: Philadelphia, 1972.

Rogers, Carl. "Carl Rogers Describes His Way of Facilitating Encounter Groups." *American Journal of Nursing*, Vol. 71 No. 2 (February, 1971), 275-279.

Scheidman, Jean. "Remotivation Without Labels." *Journal of Psychiatric and Mental Health Services*, Vol. 14 No. 7 (July, 1976), 41-42.

Swanson, Mary G. "A Check List for Group Leaders." *Perspectives in Psychiatric Care*, Vol. 3 No. 3 (1969) 120-126.

Veninga, Robert, and Fredlund, Delphie J. "Teaching the Group Approach." *Nursing Outlook*, Vol. 22 No. 6 (June, 1974), 373-376.

chapter 9

the therapeutic environment

learning objectives

On completion of this chapter, the reader should be able to:

1 Define *therapeutic environment.*
2 Identify the three significant components that contribute to the creation and maintenance of a therapeutic environment.
3 Learn specific nursing behaviors that contribute to the therapeutic environment.
4 Identify the biological, physical and psychological influences of the therapeutic environment.

A therapeutic environment is a deliberate set of immediate living situations and experiences geared toward problem solving, resolution of conflict and the implementation of stress-decreasing goals. As such, a therapeutic environment can be viewed from two perspectives—the micro environment and the macro environment. The microtherapeutic environment includes a hospital ward, doctor's office or patient's home. The macro setting—the large environment—includes the totality of any institutional facility or community in which the patient is currently residing. Broadly interpreted the therapeutic environment can encompass a patient's entire living situation, because transactions and relationships to significant others and places and objects are the outputs of the patient's frame of reference and are thereby affected by the degree of pathological dysfunction.

The essence of the therapeutic environment is the emotional, social and psychological climate prevailing within the patient's setting that allows him to focus on the resolution of existent problems and conflicts. In order to be considered therapeutic an environment must contain those factors which contribute to, provide for and promote maximum opportunity for growth and development. Nursing assumes an important function in the creation and maintainence of a therapeutic environment in that the nurse provides for healthy interactions and learning situations which enable the patient to formulate adequate adjustments.

We believe there are three major components that contribute to the formation and maintenance of a therapeutic environment. These are *privacy, safety and protection,* and *comfort.* In this chapter we explore each of these components and highlight several specific nursing activities and areas of responsibility.

The changing emphasis within the field of psychiatric-mental health nursing practice currently places priority on expanding the role of the nurse within the construct of community mental health facilities. Our primary emphasis is directed toward residential facilities, although the principles can be universally applied to any environment or setting. The nurse should apply the principles of a therapeutic environment to whatever setting patient care takes place.

privacy: a basic need

Everybody has a need for privacy. Throughout recorded history people have sought to protect this basic need for themselves, their loved ones and their immediate community. Anthropologists have vividly described the privacy sought and protected by mankind through past milleniums. As technology developed people became more social and interdependent on extended environments to provide them with the means by which they could achieve daily needs. Today the confines of privacy continue to be valued and protected.

Hospitalization interferes with the satisfactory gratification of this need, particularly in psychiatric settings where patients and their behavior are subjected to close, continuous observation by the nurse, members of the staff and other patients. Experience has taught us that large wards tend to dehumanize rather than support a sense of dignity, respect for individuality, self-worth, personal identity and privacy. Yet these are the essential elements of nursing care for individuals who are experiencing emotional and other psychological distresses. So the nurse's attention should be directed toward utilizing the physical environment to develop an atmosphere that promotes as much privacy as possible.

One of the environmental modifications the nurse should consider is the arrangement of furniture in the recreation room, common areas and visitor's rooms of the hospital wards. The furniture should be placed in small, circular or semicircular groupings, much as in a family room or living room. This type of physical arrangement provides the patient with tangible evidence that his need for privacy is recognized, acknowledged and accepted. Small groups of patients can talk together without disrupting other groups that might be in the immediate area, and a patient and his visitor can have at least some privacy.

One or two small rooms should be set aside for individual use. This provides a private area for patients whose therapeutic plan permits them to be ambulatory. Away from the general flurry of ward activities, patients can be alone, read, play their radio or musical instruments or share their experiences with special friends they have selected among other patients, without being interrupted or overheard. These small rooms could also be used by staff members for interviewing, counseling or "rapping" with the assurance of privacy during therapeutic engagements.

In our culture bathing and toileting are considered private functions. Most people are accustomed to carrying out these functions alone without assistance or supervision. It can be quite embarrassing when patients have to bathe or shower with other patients or "according to schedule." Rarely do large institutions provide a bath in each patient's room. To minimize the feelings of embarrassment and reluctance to maintain personal hygiene due to such lack of privacy, only a minimum number of personnel should be deployed to assist or supervise during bathing periods. The nurse should schedule bathing and toileting periods after examining the patient's preference and illiciting related feelings from the patient.

Personal possessions, however trivial, take on added significance when the patient is hospitalized. For the patient they become a part of his identity, contribute to his feelings of security, provide a sense of ownership and serve as a link with the reality of the environment outside the hospital. Disappearance or misplacement of personal items can produce an increase in anxiety, extend frustration and foster distrust.

Provisions must be made which guarantee the preservation and privacy of the patient's personal effects as demonstrated within this actual case history.

> Mr. Ragan a 57-year-old, divorced, male was readmitted to a state hospital following an exacerbation of his psychiatric condition diagnosed as schizophrenia, paranoid type. He had stopped taking his medications and was imbibing alcoholic beverages in order to "relax and sleep." His aged mother had died of natural causes approximately eleven months prior to admission and Mr. Ragan continued to reside alone at the parental home. Mr. Ragan had been unemployed and maintained himself with disability benefits from Social Security.
>
> One day Mr. Ragan had become intoxicated and fell asleep in a dilapidated easy chair. A fire broke out because of his careless smoking and he was miraculously saved by the alertness and swiftness of the local firemen. Subsequent to treatment for smoke inhalation at the local hospital the doctor recommended psychiatric hospitalization and treatment because the patient was confused, guarded, suspicious and hostile.
>
> Relatives reported that Mr. Ragan had been acting bizarre for some time. He did not leave the house except late at night to purchase alcohol and he refused to allow anyone to enter his home. After hospitalization, the rela-

tives discovered that the utilities had been turned off because Mr. Ragan had not paid the bills. After the fire the Health Department condemned the dwelling as unfit and unsafe for habitation. The Probate Court awarded Mr. Ragan's sister legal guardianship of his affairs. At the same time Mr. Ragan's mother's will was probated and the home was bequeathed to the patient.

Several weeks after admission Mr. Ragan was assisted in purchasing a new wardrobe since his clothing had been destroyed in the fire. Two days later, another patient stole Mr. Ragan's new clothing and absconded from the hospital. This incident intensified Mr. Ragan's suspicions, guardedness and hostility. He began to accuse the staff of collusion with his sister to keep his money and his inheritance from him. He refused to participate in ward activities and was constantly complaining about his personal dignity being "trampled on" by everyone. He was verbally hostile and made frequent collect calls to his sister in order to ventilate. Mr. Ragan would claim that everything in his life had been taken from him—his wife, mother, home, money, freedom—and insisted on leaving the hospital against medical advice.

This behavior continued for six weeks and created a series of disruptions for himself, other patients and ward activities. When Mr. Ragan was being disruptive, he would isolate himself from everyone by sitting alone in the corner of the room. Because of Mr. Ragan's limited financial benefits he was awarded a clothing voucher from the county welfare department through the collaborate efforts of the nurse and social worker. The nurse requested a special order for a lock and key to be placed on his bedside closet; she gave Mr. Ragan one key and placed a spare key in the safety of the nursing station in case Mr. Ragan would lose his key. She requested other staff persons to bring in extra hangers they might have at home to give to Mr. Ragan.

When Mr. Ragan and the nurse returned from their shopping trip there was a noted change in the patient. Smiling, he carefully placed his new clothing, new hat, new shoes and even gloves in his locker. The nurse reported that Mr. Ragan had offered to buy her lunch and coffee. His facial muscles seemed to relax and his eyes were brighter. Mr. Ragan began to attend group therapy regularly. He became gentle and courteous towards others and took great pride in personal hygiene and appearance. His appetite improved and he began to involve himself in planning for his discharge to a halfway house in the community.

Another consideration for privacy, often overlooked by the staff, is respect for closed doors. A patient's room is in a way his home away from home. Consequently, the patient is entitled to respect, courtesy, and privacy as though he were indeed in his own home. How many people do you know who go to the house next door and enter without knocking and receiving permission to enter? Yet many staff persons push open the door to a patient's room without knocking. A healthy respect for privacy does not mean allowing the patient to isolate himself from the therapeutic environment and the usual daily activities of the hospital ward. It does mean respecting the limited physical space a patient has for quiet reflection, periods of rest or uninterrupted relaxation.

Staff need privacy as much as the patients in order to execute their duties and maximize the benefits of the therapeutic environment. Daily contacts with individuals and groups whose primary problems are psychologic require a tremendous expenditure of emotional and physical energy. Thus, an area where staff can periodically retreat for readjusting their perspectives, recuperating their energy and regaining objectivity is a must. In addition, privacy is needed by staff for engaging in clinical conferences, planning patient care, sharing nursing reports and discussing relevant and sundry patient problems.

A nursing station is *not* a private place. It is the center from which the daily activities of the ward are directed and it is open on a twenty-four-hour basis. Here the nurses and other staff members are accessible to the patients, and frequently several patients at a time approach the staff for various reasons. This flurry of activity surrounding the nursing station makes it a very open and public place. Consequently, it is not an expedient setting for nurse-patient interviews or counseling. Thus, utilizing other offices and private small rooms, as described above, allows the nursing station to remain open and freely accessible to the patients at all times.

However, medication rooms are areas that require absolute privacy. For years, these rooms have been attached to nursing stations. This arrangement has some potentially undesirable effects. One is the numerous interruptions by staff or patients which interfere with the level of attention and concentration of the nurse pouring medications. This interference can possible result in errors in the distribution of patient medication. Since the pouring of medication requires diligent attention, we believe the medication room should be placed in close proximity, but not adjacent to, the nursing station and that it should be situated away from the general flow of ward traffic.

safety and protection: a necessity

Provision for patient safety and protection has always been a high priority in the nursing profession. The major emphasis is appropriately on the creation of a physical environment that meets the physiological and psychosocial needs of the patient while protecting him from injury—by self, from others or from objects. The idea of safety and protection implies a great deal, both from a physical as well as a psychological standpoint. Shatterproof windows, heavy gauge screening, locked doors and fire-fighting equipment are all important devices used to insure patient safety and protection; however, they are not wholly sufficient. The therapeutic environment can neither exist nor be effective without the provision and consideration of additional factors which influence the safety and protection of the patient.

Through hospitalization the outside community is protected from the patient. It has been our experience that nurses seldom consider the reverse implications, that is, that the nurse has an equal obligation to protect the patient from the community. By community, we mean both those within and outside the ward setting. In psychiatric-mental health settings, observation and interventive techniques are synonymous with patient care. Therefore, alertness spontaneous application with interventive techniques allow the nurse to interpret certain behavioral patterns or verbal statements by the patient that predict the patient's emotional state and his potential for physical, dangerous acting out toward himself, others or objects within his immediate environment. Thus, this type of nursing behavior, coupled with deliberate listening, can frequently lead to constructive interventions that protect a patient from himself and others.

Where locked wards are still in use, the handling of keys becomes a critical feature in creating a protective therapeutic environment. Loss, misplacement or careless handling of keys gives rise to potential hazards. When keys are lost, a search *must* be made. Searching can produce physical and psychological discomfort for patients and staff. It might result in humiliation for all; the imposition of punitive and retaliatory rules for patients; the creation of a feeling of insecurity for both patients and staff; and lastly, the possibility of loss of life to the patient and resultant guilt feelings on the part of the staff.

There are several practical solutions the nurse can employ to minimize loss or misplacement of keys. One is to enforce accountability and responsibility by use of a periodic check to see where staff are carrying their keys and by observing the kinds of habits they develop with respect to their use and proper replacement. Along with observation and fact finding goes verbal encouragement of proper respect for and use of keys. Another solution is for the nurse to set an example through her own behavior—if the nurse is careless others will be careless, if the nurse is aware and concerned so too will other staff. Careless handling includes such traumatizing habits as swinging a set of keys around the finger as the nurse walks down the hall, or wearing the keys around her neck on a ribbon or chain like a pendant, or jingling them in the pocket as she stands talking to a patient or another staff member. These habits are psychologically injurious to patients in that the nonverbal behavior demonstrates a lack of respect, and in the eyes of the patient, the staff member is placed in the position of a "jailer" as opposed to a helping and caring person. Such behavior by the nurse or any other staff member openly invites abusive behavior. It may take the form of personal attack, resulting in injury to self and others, or it may be in the form of resisting other rules or regulations. In either case, physical and psychological trauma is produced for the patient and staff alike.

Another aspect conducive to the creation of a protective environment is the placement of emergency equipment. All emergency equipment should be strategically located and in sufficient amounts to meet the needs of the unit. The equipment should be accessible to all levels of personnel, and all ward personnel should be able to demonstrate efficient performance of necessary procedures related to the use of this equipment. This emergency equipment must be in good working order at all times. One major benefit for staff of this kind of preparedness is that as staff become more secure in the knowledge of their ability to handle emergency situations, they will be more relaxed and demonstrate a decreased level of anxiety. Patients benefit from the staff's knowledge and preparedness in two ways: first, through direct, effective, efficient, nursing care management in an emergency situation; and second, through a generalized feeling of increased comfort, confidence and reliability of staff to deal with the unexpected.

The following is an account of an actual incident that occurred in a psychiatric center at the time this chapter was being written. This case illustrates the vital importance of the maintenance and use of emergency equipment in a psychiatric-mental health setting. It also clearly points out the nurse's obligation to assume responsibility for applying the concepts of protection and safety to every facet of patient care.

Mr. Richards is a 69-year-old, single, Caucasian male who has been hospitalized at a psychiatric center for several years for treatment of crystallized process schizophrenia.

His physical deterioration was evident by his stooped shoulders, high-stepping gait, total disregard for personal hygiene and appearance and, while he was not recalcitrant, the nursing staff had to repeat everything to him many times before he showed any signs of comprehension. He wore eye glasses on the tip of his nose and would bend his head forward to see. He wore dentures. Both these prothesis were often forgotten or misplaced.

On this day, Mr. Richards was eating a lunch of Polish sausage and potato salad. One of the nurses observed him choking and holding his throat. She immediately alerted the other staff while running to the patient. The Heimlich technique was not effective and food particles were manually pulled from the throat. It was then observed that Mr. Richards had tried to swallow solid food without masticating because he did not have his dentures. When the doctor ordered an airway, the nurse discovered that there was none on the unit. The ambu bag had a hole in it and the two oxygen tanks were not functioning. Both these items were requested from another unit. By the time they arrived the patient was unconscious. An emergency tracheotomy was performed and the patient was transferred to the intensive care unit in critical condition.

Another hazard to which patients are exposed is the presence of strangers on the ward. The nurse must be aware of their presence and the reason for their being there. The nurse must insist on immediate notification, be they plumber, consulting physician, cleaning person, volunteer or visitor. Each category of "stranger" that enters the ward setting poses a potential threat to patient welfare and demands that the nurse intervene on behalf of the patients. If a plumber comes, for example, the nurse should inform the team member assigned to close observation of a potentially suicidal patient and alert him to possible self-injurious agents of a plumber's equipment like poisonous drain cleaning powder or sharp pieces of metal that could be used as a knife. If a consulting physician comes, the nurse would need to know if the patient was informed of the consultation and is available to be seen; also the nurse would need to speak with the physician and relate any pertinent data he may require as well as be available to receive any important instructions on the orders he writes. If a visitor comes, the nurse would want to carefully and courteously instruct the individual regarding the rules and regulations of the ward, not only with respect to those which apply to their particular family member or friend but also, those which apply to the ward in general.

The development and maintenance of a therapeutic environment in terms of protection also requires that the nurse pay attention to such minute details as having an adequate number of ash trays conveniently located; clean and serviced drinking fountains; proper ventilation; fire regulations posted; periodic fire drills conducted for staff and patients; toilet paper holders, paper towel and soap dispensers refilled. In such a constantly changing place as a ward, the creation of a protective environment is no easy task. It requires that the nurse exercise constant vigilance and judgment.

comfort: a right

To be therapeutic, the environment must be comfortable physically and psychologically. To achieve a satisfactory and healthy level of comfortableness, the nurse should create an appealing aesthetic atmosphere, provide for monitoring biological functions, and foster emotional growth and development.

The provision for comfort as part of a therapeutic environment includes measures to satisfactorily monitor biological functioning. Because an individual's primary diagnosis and reason for hospitalization falls in the area of an identifiable psychological problem, the physiological aspects of the total person may be de-emphasized and sometimes even completely overlooked. The nurse must keep in mind that treatment and care of any patient, regardless of diagnosis, includes the soma and the psyche as an integrated whole. Although she may not need to care for a recognized health deficiency, she should do preventative health care and health teaching. It is important to realize the impact emotional and psychological distress has on physiological functioning. In both schizophrenia and depression, for example, food intake may have a profound effect. Concentration or avoidance of certain foods may produce severe diarrhea or constipation, resulting in electrolyte imbalance which in turn may produce signs and symptoms similar to known side effects of tranquilizing agents. Until attention is paid to biological monitoring, the nurse has no factual data on which to differentiate possible causes. It is only after the differentiation has been made that the nurse can institute appropriate intervention.

Another example that points out the necessity for monitoring biological functioning is the importance of taking the temperature when there are specific drug combinations and climatic conditions. This is particularly true when thorazine and cogentin are given together. Both drugs affect the heat regulating function of the hypothalmus. In hot, humid weather the patient is susceptible to heat prostration because this combination of drugs prevents him from perspiring adequately. The only way the nurse can make sure the patient is not experiencing temperature irregularities is by monitoring.

Our biological nature exists in accordance with definitive patterns but each individual's pattern is different. There is for each person a specific, constant biological rhythm and timing—biorhythm. Illness or stress does not necessarily change the rhythm or timing but it does interefere with its regularity. This interference accounts for some of the increase in the level of anxiety and feelings of discomfort expressed by patients as somatic complaints.

Many of these complaints are, in fact, due to the loss of synchronization in the person's biological functioning. To prevent such disruption, it is important for the nurse to learn as much as possible about the normal life pattern of each individual.

The gathering of this factual information should occur immediately or as soon after admission as possible. (See Chapter 21 for assessment and the development of the nursing care plan.) The patient is the prime source for this information; however, if the person is unable to supply data regarding self, then relatives, friends, and acquaintances of the patient should be contacted. Assessment of biological functioning is as vital as the assessment of social, cultural or psychological functioning in determining and evaluating deviations. Individual biological functioning must be considered when planning nursing care. Some individuals function adequately on six hours of sleep while others require ten hours. If we believe that nursing care is based on individual needs, then it becomes imperative to adapt usual ward routines to accommodate individual functioning. Thus, consideration should be given to such things as the scheduling of activities. Activities should be at a time when the patient is most alert and receptive. Adaptation to meet individual patient needs does not imply that the unit functions chaotically. Any large system such as a hospital has to operate on some type of organized structure, but structure should be flexible and humane rather than rigid, impersonal and dogmatic in its rules and regulations. There must be built into the system the attitude that the individual comes first and that the preservation of the system takes second place.

The therapeutic environment can promote comfort by fostering emotional growth and development. Since the therapeutic process is one of reeducation, the setting of the unit must incorporate and utilize those features most likely to be found in the majority of social living situations. Inclusion of such elements encourages feelings of identity, security, independence, self-actualization and reality orientation. If these factors of growth and development are to be realized, the nurse must pay special attention to the details involved in any usual living experience. For instance, we are a time-oriented society; but hospitalized individuals tend to lose track of time and may even manifest time disorientation. Some simple, practical aids for the nurse to use in dealing with this problem are clocks, calendars and daily newspapers. Convenient placement and accessibility to these aids encourages independent functioning. Their use decreases the need for patients to ask the staff the time or the date, and decreases labeling a patient as confused or disoriented. The decrease in interruptions gives staff more time to communicate with patients on a more in-depth level of therapeutic interaction.

Another environmental factor influencing growth and development concerns the personal possessions of patients. We are a materialistic society. We closely identify who we are with what we have. Personal possessions are an extension of ourselves. As such, they play an important part in the development and maintenance of our identity as individuals. Hospitalization forces people to limit the number and types of possessions they can keep with them. Therefore, those which they have take on an even greater significance.

Nursing has paid lip service to the need for the nurse to develop an attitude of acceptance toward the patient. Unfortunately, nursing has sometimes become caught up in hospital bureaucracy. The result is that the patient is subjected to a dehumanizing experience. The idea of a therapeutic environment implies that the health team limit the restrictions imposed on all specific components which comprise the whole person. Personal possessions are one such component. They reflect a person's social, cultural, economic and religious status. They convey to the observer how and in what manner the individual has established his interdependency within society. When a person is deprived of a significant portion of himself, the health team is also deprived. Assessment and identification of problem areas, and the establishment of guidelines for normalcy for a particular individual is impaired because a significant portion of that person is not available for observation, evaluation and incorporation into the total treatment program.

Personal possessions include a variety of items which have often been viewed in the past as either nonessential, too costly to be safe from light-fingered individuals, superfluous or potentially hazardous. Items which have been accorded these designations are personal wearing apparel, cosmetics, wedding and engagement rings, costume jewelry, purses, wallets, ties, nostalgic mementoes and souvenirs, a favorite chair, needlework, musical instruments, family pictures and projects completed in occupational therapy. To insure psychological comfort and facilitate the growth and development processes with respect to personal possessions, the nurse should carefully examine existing hospital policy and work toward offering modifications where the restrictions are excessively limiting. Another nursing action is to discuss with the patient the meaning various personal items have for him. If it is determined that the significance is great, the nurse should make every attempt to carry out her advocacy role and provide him with the "security blanket" he needs. Other ways to advocate for a therapeutic environment in fostering growth and development might be to encourage participation in ward government; invite the patient to assume a co-responsibility with staff for effecting changes within his environment; set up and maintain ward kitchens to which patients have free access to make a pot of tea, bake a cake or make some popcorn; provide places for patients to visit with their children; organize groups of patients to concentrate on beautification of hospital grounds; introduce a ward pet; and as many more modifications or adaptations as the nurse can think of—the possibilities are endless.

Comfort is an all-encompassing multifaceted concept that requires thoughtful consideration and attentiveness by the nurse. Some very common aspects of daily living which are frequently overlooked include such necessary items as a bed with a matress that is whole, free from odors and not sagging. Sufficient bed linen, including sheets that are not torn, and pillow cases, blankets and spreads are also important. How often have you awakened in the morning and put your feet on the cold floor? This is discomforting. It often fosters the reluctance of the patient to arise quickly or even when necessary during the night—slippers might help.

Bathing requires towels and wash cloths. The nurse creates patient comfort by seeing to it that these bathing items are readily available for use.

Also, such daily items as shampoos, soap, shaving equipment, hair spray, nail clippers, nail files, aftershave lotion, deodorants, hand and body lotion should be available to the patient. This does not mean that the institution must provide these items, but that the nurse assumes responsibility for contacting family members or relatives to supply such items. Where there are no family resources the nurse should advocate for patient needs to the appropriate agencies both within and without the care setting, such as The Red Cross, volunteer services, church groups and welfare offices.

Another aspect of comfort involves wearing apparel. Whenever possible patients should be encouraged to wear their own clothes. If they do, the nurse should make certain that the clothing is appropriate to the season, intact, coordinated and that the total appearance of the patient is neat, clean and presentable. Where the patient must rely on the institution to provide these items, the nurse must insist on advocating in the patient's behalf for correct sizes, sufficient numbers to allow for changing, and up-to-date style and fashion. For too long, institutions have been allowed to singularly dehumanize and perpetuate the worst image of mental patients with personal apparel that approximates the medieval ages or the scarecrow in the corn field. It is time for the nursing profession to realize that we are now in the twentieth century, post Dorothea Dix, and that we live in the age of advocacy and human psychology.

An additional area of concern in the maintenance of a therapeutic environment is the creation of an aesthetic atmosphere because of its important influence and impact on both behavior and feeling. Where possible, in selecting color schemes, one factor the nurse must consider is the type of resident population: the potential age range of the population as well as the predominant sex of the occupants. For example, pink walls, draperies and spreads would usually be considered unsuitable for male patients, whereas female patients would generally find them very acceptable.

Another factor the nurse should consider in selecting appropriate color schemes is the effect color has on mood. Dark colors can tend to be oppressive and create a feeling of gloom and dejection. These colors then, certainly would not be suitable for individuals who are exhibiting symptoms of depression. Soft, warm, light colors tend to create an atmosphere which aids in promoting a feeling of comfort and well-being. On the other hand, overly bright hues and shades may produce negative effects by exposing an individual to overstimulation. Color or lack of it can make a working or living environment very pleasant or very negative and uncomfortable.

It seems to be almost a universal policy that when a unit is painted, everything—the walls, the moldings, the doors, the doorways, etc.—gets painted in the same color. The nurse must assume responsibility for making suggestions about the kinds of colors used as well as providing for individuality in the painting. The nurse can accomplish this by seeing to it that different areas of the unit are painted in different colors. The choice of color depends on the purpose for which the room is to be used and the needs and desires of its perspective occupants. A blending of colors and motifs creates an environment which reflects a consideration for the humanity of patients and staff.

In addition to color, proportion and design are also important in produc-

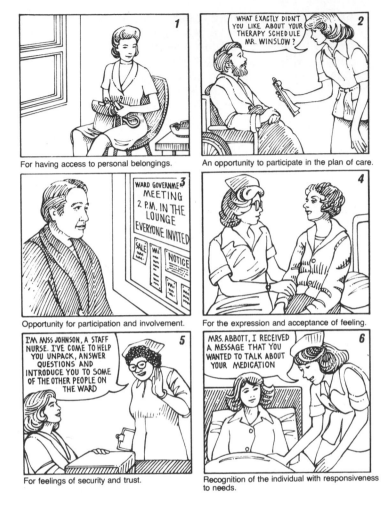

Figure 9-1

ing an appealing aesthetic atmosphere. By proportion we mean the dimensions used, that is, the size and ratio of such things as room space, furniture, draperies, pictures and other furnishings. Living space in terms of room size is a necessary element for consideration in planning for a therapeutic environment if the freedom "to move" and "to be" is to be encouraged and maintained. In planning the amount of space needed, thought should be given to the purpose for which the room is to be used; the type and size of furniture and/or equipment it is to accommodate, as well as, the possible maximum number of people it will be required to hold. A light background gives a sharper outline. Smaller furniture increases the size of the room. Cramped quarters for patients and staff tends to produce inhibitory effects and is therefore not conducive to productive functioning or to the develop-

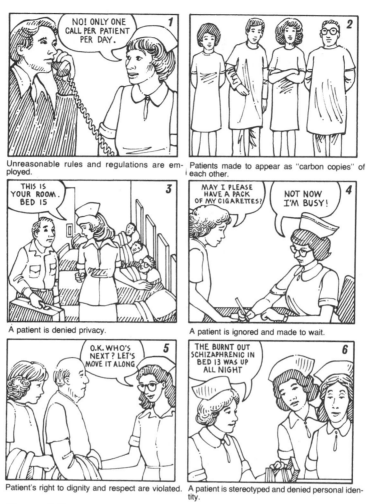

Figure 9-2

ment of a feeling of freedom of movement. All too often, furnishings are purchased in bulk lots and selected only on the basis of their utilitarian value. Where possible, furnishings should be selected on the basis of their size, suitability and appropriateness for the area in which they will be used.

There are other features which contribute to the creation of an aesthetic environment. One example is the use of table cloths, attractive china, glassware and table arrangements in the dining room. Objects pleasing to the eye do much for the promotion of comfort. They also create an atmosphere in which positive expectations are directed toward acceptable social behavior. Other important items are the introduction of such things as pictures, mirrors, plants, carpeting in living areas and toss pillows. These additions contribute to comfort by making the ward atmosphere more livable and homelike as opposed to the dreary, gloomy, sterile atmosphere which still prevails in many wards. The creation of this kind of "design for living" falls within the province of nursing. The nurse is responsible for using her creativity and perceptiveness to advocate and recommend those features which contribute to the maintenance of an environment that is pleasing, appropriate and useful.

In summary, this chapter has pointed out some of the significant factors involved in the creation and maintenance of a therapeutic environment. We have identified the major components which must be considered: *privacy, safety and protection* and *comfort*. In each of these categories we have emphasized specific nursing activities that are essential, which when utilized and integrated can produce an environment conducive to healthy functioning and which stimulate the patient to assume an active, participatory role in the psychotherapeutic processes of his treatment.

suggested readings

Alfano, Genrose J. "Healing or Caretaking—Which Will It Be?" *Nursing Clinics of North America,* Vol. 6 No. 2 (June, 1971), 273-280.

Almond, Richard. *The Healing Community: Dynamics of The Therapeutic Milieu.* Jason Aronson: New York, 1974.

Bunning, Erwin. *The Physiological Clock.* 2d ed. Springer-Verlag: New York, Inc.: New York, 1967.

Colquhoun, W. P., ed. *Biological Rhythms and Human Performance.* Academic Press, Inc.: New York, 1971.

Dienemann, Jackie. "The Application of Psychotherapeutic Conceptual Models in Nursing Practice." *Journal of Psychiatric Nursing and Mental Health Service,* Vol. 14 No. 5 (May, 1976), 28-30.

Emde, N. Robert. "Limiting Regression in the Therapeutic Community." *American Journal of Nursing,* Vol. 67 No. 5 (May, 1967), 1010.

Grant, Donna Allen, and Klell, Cynthia. "For Goodness Sake—Let Your Patient Sleep!" *Nursing '74,* Vol. 4 No. 11 (November, 1974), 54-57.

Hall, Beverly A. "Mutual Withdrawal: The Non-Participant in a Therapeutic Community." *Perspectives in Psychiatric Care,* Vol. 14 No. 2 (1976) 75-77:93.

Hayes, Joyce Samhammer. "The Psychiatric Nurse as Sociotherapist." *American Journal of Nursing,* Vol. 62 No. 6 (June, 1962), 64-67.

Holmes, Marguerite, and Werner, Jean. *Psychiatric Nursing in a Therapeutic Community.* MacMillan Company: New York, 1967.

Jones, Maxwell, M.D. *The Therapeutic Community, a Treatment Method in Psychiatry.* Basic Books, Inc.: New York, 1953.

Kinchsloe, Marsha. "Democratization in the Therapeutic Community." *Perspectives in Psychiatric Care,* Vol. 11 No. 2 (1973), 75-79.

Kraft, Alan M. "The Therapeutic Community." *American Handbook of Psychiatry.* 2d ed. Edited by Silvan Arieti. Vol. III. Russell Sage Foundation: New York, 1966, 542-551.

Kramer, Marlene, and Schmalenberg, Claudia. *Path to Biculturalism.* Contemporary Publishing, Inc.: Wakefield, Massachusetts. 1977.

Kukuk, Helen M. "Safety Precautions: Protecting Your Patients and Yourself." *Nursing 76,* Vol. 6 No. 5 (May, 1976), 45-51.

————. "Safety Precautions: Protecting Your Patients and Yourself." *Nursing 76,* Vol. 6 No. 6 (June, 1976), 49-52.

Laing, Mary M., Murphy, Patricia L., and Schultz, Ellen D. "The Planning and Implementation of a Psychiatric Self-Care Unit." *Journal of Psychiatric and Mental Health Services,* Vol. 15 No. 7 (July, 1977), 30-34.

Lewis, Alfred B., and Selzer, Michael. "Some Neglected Issues in Milieu Therapy." *Hospital and Community Psychiatry,* Vol. 23 No. 10 (October, 1972).

Mitchell, Ross. "The Therapeutic Community." In *Psychiatric–Mental Health Nursing: Contemporary Readings,* edited by Backer, Barbara A., Dubbert, Patricia M. and Eisenman, Elaine. J. P. D. Van Nostrand Co., Inc.: New York, 1978, 377-382.

Natalini, John J. "The Human Body as a Biological Clock." *American Journal of Nursing,* Vol. 77 No. 7 (July, 1977), 1130-1132.

Robertson, Patricia A. "The Therapeutic Community and the Nurse: A Blurring of Traditional Roles." *Journal of Psychiatric Nursing and Mental Health Services,* Vol. 14 No. 4 (April, 1976), 28-31.

Ryan, John L. "The Single Room: A Right for Every Patient's Privacy." *Nursing Digest* (September-October, 1975), 46-47.

Schwartz, Morris S., and Shockley, Emmy Lanning. *The Nurse and The Mental Patient.* John Wiley & Sons, Inc.: New York, 1956.

Siegel, Nathaniel H. "What is a Therapeutic Community?" In *Psychiatric Nursing— Developing Psychiatric Nursing Skills, Vol. I.* edited by Dorothy Mereness. Wm. C. Brown Co. Publishers: Dubuque, Iowa, 1966, 283-288.

Stevens, Leonard F. "What Makes a Ward Climate Therapeutic?" In *Psychiatric Nursing—Developing Psychiatric Nursing Skills, Vol. I.* Edited by Dorothy Mereness. Wm. C. Brown Co. Publishers: Dubuque, Iowa, 1966, 289-292.

Wilson, Holly Skodol. "Limiting Intrusion—Social Control of Outsiders in a Healing Community." *Nursing Research,* Vol. 26 No. 2 (March/April, 1977), 103-111.

part 2

chapter 10

developmental theories— a frame of reference

learning objectives

On completion of this chapter the reader should be able to:

1 Identify the major contributions made by Freud, Sullivan, Erikson and Piaget to developmental theory.
2 Recognize the stages of normal growth and development.
3 Identify the stages of development conceived by Freud, Sullivan, Erikson and Piaget.
4 Understand the significance of developmental theory in the practice of psychiatric nursing.

People are complex social creatures. An individual is a composite of all he is, all that he thinks, feels and does both consciously and unconsciously. He is the product of his experiences which he has integrated through the five basic senses—sight, hearing, touch, taste and smell. He is like all others and yet he remains distinctly individual. A person functions from his personal framework, and all his component parts—mind, body and spirit—work in unison to produce and maintain equilibrium. Hence, there are interrelationships among the phsyical, intellectual, social, spiritual and emotional components of the self.

The individual is engaged in an ongoing interactional process with his environment which facilitates movement toward continued growth and development. His total functioning is an outcome of his developmental process—the quantitative and qualitative ways in which the individual changes over time. His personality with its intrinsic dignity is a reflection of his composite nature and as such reveals his instincts, needs, desires, physical talents and attributes, feelings, beliefs and values. He manifests the characteristics of his personality through his verbal and nonverbal communication and through his behavioral patterns.

A working knowledge of fundamental concepts and theories of human development is essential if the nurse is to arrive at an understanding of human functioning and ultimately interpret a person's behavior in light of the developmental process. This knowledge gives the nurse a frame of reference upon which to begin to assess where the patient is within his life experience. The nurse's application of this knowledge results in the delivery of competent and comprehensive nursing care.

Psychiatric nursing predicates its practice on the assumption of an eclectic approach which combines the psychoanalytic, interpersonal and social theories with learning theory. We have briefly summarized the contributions made by Freud, Sullivan, Erikson and Piaget to assist the student to establish a frame of reference and to rapidly review some major concepts relevant to each of these developmental theories.

major theories

Within the field of human development there are a multiplicity of diverse and controversial theories. For simplification, these theories may be broadly divided into four major schools of thought: the psychoanalytic, the interpersonal, the social and the cognitive.

Analytic theory and the first systematic theories of development came from the research and writings of Sigmund Freud. From this initial thrust the analytic school of thought was expanded and the first Freudians—Jung, Adler, Rank, Meyer and Ferencz—made significant contributions. Each of these theorists expanded the basic Freudian theories by adding different dimensions and placing varying degrees of emphasis on the growth and developmental process. Basically, analytic theory views man and his development as an intraphysic experience related to the satisfaction and gratification of basic needs and drives.

From this foundation came the Neo-Freudian groups that integrated the psychic process with interpersonal transactions. With the advent of interpersonal theory, whose advocates include Sullivan, Horney and Fromm, there was gradual movement away from viewing the unconscious as the prime motivator of human behavior. In essence, interpersonal theory focuses on the kind of relationship an individual establishes and maintains with a "significant other."

Subsequently, social theory, an outgrowth and expansion of interpersonal theory, was advanced through the efforts of such people as Eric Erikson and Kurt Lewin. The chief concept underlying social theory is the humanistic, realistic and conscious development of the individual's personality as a direct outcome of a group interactional process.

Each of these schools of thought contributed ideas of personality development in terms of an individual's biophysical, psychological and social growth. Within this theoretical framework, however, little emphasis is placed on the cognitive development of the individual. Concurrently, but not relatedly, behavioral psychologists such as Hull, Skinner and Piaget advanced theories of the development of cognitive styles and motor skill ability in relationship to the development of learning theory.

Table 10-1 is a brief description of the major theories and contributions made by Freud, Sullivan, Erikson and Piaget. Table 10-2 illustrates the stages of development postulated by each of these theorists.

In comparing Freud's, Sullivan's, Erikson's and Piaget's conceptualizations about the developmental process, it can be noted that although they differ regarding time span, specific aspects of development and emphasis within a particular stage, each theory accounts for a complete process. Thus, regardless of which theory the nurse uses as her frame of reference, certain outcomes are expected and should occur in the developmental process. In other words, each individual must move through a series of operations—physical, mental, emotional and social—which lead to maturation, even though the rate of movement may be different for each individual. All stages need to be completed if the individual is to progress. Illness or deviation occurs when progression is inhibited, interrupted or terminated. Successful completion of the developmental process requires that the individual be able to:

1 Express primary needs and feelings.
2 Learn to count on others for part of his need gratification and fulfillment.
3 Recognize people and objects as being external to self.
4 Develop an ego identity.
5 Accept delayed gratification.
6 Develop, refine and coordinate physical skills.
7 Establish, integrate and utilize a set of values.
8 Function independently.
9 Use cooperation and compromise in dealing with others.
10 Pursue intellectual and aesthetic activities.
11 Engage in heterosexual relationships.
12 Develop an intimate relationship.
13 Establish a work role.
14 Adapt to changing roles.
15 Attain self-actualization.

TABLE 10-1
A COMPARISON OF THE MAJOR THEORETICAL CONTRIBUTIONS OF FREUD, SULLIVAN, ERIKSON AND PIAGET

Sigmund Freud (1856-1939)	Harry Stack Sullivan (1892-1949)	Eric Erikson	Jean Paul Piaget
1) First to identify and classify developmental stages.	1) First to focus on the interactional process between mother and child.	1) First to include adulthood as a stage of growth and focus on the formation of personal identity as a key concept.	1) First to be concerned with the development of cognition.
2) Theory focused on the concept of libidinal energy and instinctual drives as the forces which motivate behavior.	2) Theory focused on the concept of anxiety as the dynamic force in the developmental process.	2) Theory combines Freud's biological or heredity factors with Sullivan's social factors.	2) The theory concentrates on the development of intellectual capabilities with little reference to emotional or social development.
3) Developed the concept that the mind operates on three levels—the unconscious, the preconscious and the conscious. Emphasis placed on intrapsychic behavior.	3) Used Freud's concept of the unconscious and conscious mind. Emphasis placed on observable behavior.	3) Used Freud's concept of the divisions of the mind. Emphasis placed on the individual's relationship as influenced by the family, peers and society.	3) Emphasized the dual process of assimilation and accommodation with respect to the development of reasoning, language, intelligence, and the concepts of nature, time, space and causality.
4) Experience is always viewed in relation to unconscious material and reconstruction of the past.	4) Experience is viewed as an interactional process existing between self and others, which depends on previous experience.	4) Experience is viewed as a dichotomy established between basic attitudinal values and feelings.	4) Experience is viewed as a building-block process for the expansion of intrinsic capabilities.
5) The mind has a structural division—the id, the ego and the superego.	5) Experience is divided into three cognitive modes—prototaxic, parataxic, and syntaxic.	5) The extended social experience is the primary framework in learning.	5) Development is influenced by individual differences and social influences; focus is on the mind rather than on the self.

TABLE 10-1 (continued)

Sigmund Freud (1856-1939)	Harry Stack Sullivan (1892-1949)	Eric Erikson	Jean Paul Piaget
6) Developed theories while working with pathological adults, primarily neurotics.	6) Developed theories while working with pathological adults, primarily schizophrenics.	6) Developed theories while working with children and emphasized both health and illness in the personality.	6) Developed theories while working with normal, healthy children.
7) Believed that no behavioral change can be effected without understanding the content and meaning of the individual's unconscious.	7) Believed that change occurs only when improved interpersonal relationships are combined with an understanding of the basic good-bad influences.	7) Believed that behavioral change occurs only when the individual achieves integration of aptitudes, libido and social roles to form a stronger ego identity.	7) Believed that change occurs as an outcome of the socialization process.
8) Focused on emotional development.	8) Focused on emotional and interpersonal development.	8) Focused on emotional, interpersonal and spiritual development.	8) Focused on intellectual and psychomotor skill development.

TABLE 10-2

A COMPARISON OF THE DEVELOPMENT STAGES POSTULATED BY FREUD, SULLIVAN, ERICKSON AND PIAGET

Freud	Sullivan	Erikson	Piaget

I) Oral Stage (0-18 months)
a) The mouth is a source of satisfaction.
b) Two Phases:
  1) Passive
    Only interests are satisfying hunger and *sucking*
    Completely helpless, *security* is the greatest need.
    Narcissistic and egocentric, operates on *pleasure principle.*
    Omnipotent feelings are prevalent.
  2) Active
    Biting is a mode of pleasure.
    Continuous experimentation and associations.
    Sensory discriminations.
    Differentiation be-
	I) Infancy (0-18 months)
	a) The mouth is a source of satisfaction.
	b) Mouth—takes in (sucking), cuts off (biting), and pushes out (spitting) objects introduced by others.
	c) Crying, babbling and cooing are modes of communication used by the infant to call attention of adults to self.
	d) *Satisfaction response* (PLEASURE PRINCIPLE)
	Infant's biological needs are met and a mutual feeling of comfort and fulfillment is experienced by mother and child. (Mother gives and child takes.)
	e) *Empathic observation*
	Capacity to perceive feelings of others as his own immediate
		I) Oral-sensory Stage (0-12 months)
		a) The mouth is a source of satisfaction and a means of dealing with anxiety producing situations.
		b) Focus is on the development of the *basic attitudes of trust vs. mistrust.*
		c) Attitudes are formed through mother's reaction to infant needs.
			I) Sensorimotor Stage (0-12 months)
			a) Emphasis in on *preverbal intellecutal* development.
			b) Learns relationships with external objects.
			c) Focus is on physical development with gradual increase in ability to think and use language.

TABLE 10-2 (continued)

Freud	Sullivan	Erikson	Piaget
	tween mental images and reality. Differentiation of others and discovery of self. f) *Autistic invention* State of symbol activity in which the infant feels he is master of all he surveys. g) Experimentation, exploration and manipulation are methods used to acquaint self with environment.		
II) Anal Stage (1½-3 years) a) Primary activity is on learning muscular control association with urination and defecation. (*toilet training period*) b) Exhibits more self control; walks, talks, dresses and undresses c) *Negativism*—assertion of independence. d) Introduction of *reality principle, ego development.*	II) Childhood (1½-6 years) a) Begins with the capacity for communicating through speech and ends with a beginning need for association with peers. b) Uses *language* as a tool to communicate wishes and needs. c) Anus is power tool used to give or withhold a part of self to control significant people in his environment.	II) Anal-muscular Stage (1-3 years) a) Learns the extent to which the *environment* can be influenced by direct manipulation. b) Focuses on the development of the *basic attitudes of autonomy vs shame and doubt.* c) Exerts self-control and will power.	II) Preoperational Stage (2-7 years) a) Learns to use *symbols and language.* b) Learns to *imitate* and play. c) Displays *egocentricity.* d) Engages in *animistic thinking*—endowment of objects with power and ability.

TABLE 10-2 (continued)

Freud	Sullivan	Erikson	Piaget
e) Superego begins to develop. f) Engages in *parallel play*.	d) Emergence and integration of *self-concept and reflected appraisal of significant persons*. e) Awareness that postponing or delaying gratification of own wishes may bring satisfaction. f) Begins to find limits in experimentation, exploration and manipulation. g) More aggressive. h) Uses parallel play and curiosity to explore environment. i) Uses exhibitionism and mastubatory activity to become acquainted with self and others. j) Demonstrates a beginning ability to think abstractly.		

TABLE 10-2 (continued)

Freud	Sullivan	Erikson	Piaget
III) Phallic Stage (3-6 years) a) *Libidinal energy focus on the genitals.* b) Learns *sexual identity.* c) *Superego becomes internalized.* d) *Sibling rivalry* and manipulation of parents occurs. e) Intellectual and motor facilities are refined. f) Increased socialization and *associative play.*		III) Genital-locomotor Stage (3-6 years) a) Learns the extent to which being *assertive* will influence the environment. b) Focus is on the development of the *basic attitudes of initiative vs. guilt.* c) Explores the world with senses, thoughts and imagination. d) Activities demonstrate direction and purpose. e) Engages in first real social contacts through *cooperative play.* f) *Develops conscience.*	
IV) Latency (6-12 years) a) *Quiet stage* in which sexual development lies dormant, emotional tension eases. b) *Normal homosexual phase* For boys, gangs	III) Juvenile Stage (6-9 years) a) Learns to form satisfactory relationship with peers. b) *Peer norms* prevail over family norms. c) Engages in *competi-*	IV) Latency (6-12 years) a) Learns to utilize energy to create, develop and manipulate. b) Focus is on the development of *basic attitudes of industry vs. inferiority.*	III) Concrete operations Stage (7-11 years) a) Deals with visible concrete objects and relationships. b) Increased intellectual and conceptual development—employs

TABLE 10-2 (continued)

Freud	Sullivan	Erikson	Piaget
For girls, cliques c) Increased intellectual capacity. d) Starts school. e) *Identifies with teachers and peers.* f) Weakening of home ties. g) Recognizes authority figures outside home, age of *hero worship.*	*tion, experimentation,* exploration and manipulation. d) Able to cooperate and *compromise.* e) Demonstrates capacity to love. f) Distinguishes fantasy from reality. g) Exerts internal control over behavior. IV) Preadolescence (9-12 years) a) Learns to relate to a friend of the same sex—*chum relationship.* b) Concerned with group success and derives satisfaction from group accomplishment. c) Shows signs of *rebellion*—restlessness hostility, irritability. d) Assumes less responsibility for own actions. e) Moves from egocentricity to a more full social state.	c) Able to initiate and complete tasks. d) Understands rules and regulations. e) Displays *competence* and *productivity.*	*logic* and *reasoning.* c) More socialized and rule conscious.

TABLE 10-2 (continued)

Freud	Sullivan	Erikson	Piaget
	f) Uses experimentation, exploration, manipulation. g) Seeks *consensual validation* from peers.		IV) Formal Operations Stage (11-15 years) a) Develops *true abstract thought.* b) Formulates hypothesis and applies logical tests. c) *Conceptual independence.*
V) Genital Stage (12-Early Adulthood) a) Appearance of secondary sex characteristics, *reawakening of sex drives.* b) Increased concern over physical appearance. c) Strives toward *independence.* d) Development of *sexual maturity.* e) *Identity crisis.* f) Identification of love object of opposite sex. g) Intellectual Maturity. h) Plans future.	V) Early Adolescence (12-14 years) a) Experience physiological changes. b) Uses rebellion to gain Independence. c) Fantasizes, over-identifies with heroes. d) Discovers and begins relationships with opposite sex. e) Demonstrate *heightened levels of anxiety* in most interpersonal relationships.	V) Puberty and Adolescence (12-18 years) a) Demonstrates an ability to *integrate life experiences.* b) Focus is on the development of the *basic attitudes of identity vs. role diffusion.* c) Seeks partner of the opposite sex. d) Begins to establish his identity and place in society.	

131

TABLE 10-2 (continued)

Freud	Sullivan	Erikson	Piaget
	VI) Late Adolescence (14-21 years) a) Establishes an enduring intimate relationship with one member of the opposite sex. b) Self-concept becomes stabilized. c) Attains physical maturity. d) Develops ability to use logic and abstract concepts.	VI) Young Adulthood (18-25 years) a) Primarily concerned with developing an *intimate relationship* with another adult. b) Focus is on the development of the basic *attitudes of intimacy and solidarity vs. isolation.*	
	VII) Adulthood (21 years +) a) Assumes *responsibility* relevant to station in life. b) *Maintains balance and involvement* between self, family and community. c) Further develops *creativity.* d) *Reaffirms values in* life.	VII) Adulthood (25-45 years) a) Primarily concerned with establishing and maintaining a family. b) Focus is on the development of the basic *attitudes of generativity vs. stagnation.* c) Displays a marked degree of creativity. d) Adjust to circumstances of middle age. e) *Re-evaluates life's accomplishments and goals.*	

TABLE 10-2 (continued)

Freud	Sullivan	Erikson	Piaget
		VIII) Maturity (older than 45 years) a) *Acceptance of life style as meaningful and fulfilling.* b) *Focus is on the development of basic attitudes of ego integrity vs. despair.* c) Remains optimistic and continues to grow. d) Adjusts to limitations. e) Adjusts to retirement. f) Adjusts to reorganized family patterns. g) Adjusts to losses. h) Accepts death with serenity.	

Effective nursing care stems from the nurse's application of a basic principle fundamental to the developmental process, which is, that *all behavior has meaning, can be understood, and is relative to an individual's culture, specific situation and time frame.* The field of psychiatric nursing relies heavily on the use of this principle and the various theories regarding normal human development. Armed with this knowledge the nurse is in a position to recognize disruptions and disfunction within the developmental pattern, identify missing steps within the growth process and as a result, emphasize the healthy aspects while including within the plan of care those corrective experiences that may be necessary to foster further growth and promote continued development.

suggested readings

Ackerman, Nathan W. *The Psychodynamics of Family Therapy.* New York: Basic Books Inc., 1958.

Dodson, Fitzhugh. *How to Parent.* New American Library: New York, 1971.

Erickson, Eric. *Childhood and Society.* 2d ed. W. W. Norton Company: New York, 1963.

Engelhardt, Kay. "Piaget: A Prescriptive Theory For Parents." *Nursing Digest* (November-December, 1974), 22-26.

Fraiberg, Selma H. *The Magic Years.* Charles Scribner's Sons: New York, 1959.

Ginott, Haim. *Between Parent and Child.* MacMillan Publishing Company: New York, 1965.

Ginott, Haim. *Between Parent and Teenager.* MacMillan Publishing Company: New York, 1969.

Goodman, Paul. *Growing Up Absurd.* Vintage Books: New York, 1960.

Holmes, Douglas; Holmes, Monica Bychowski; and Appignanesi, Lisa. *The Language of Trust.* Science House, Inc.: 1971.

Johnston, Maxine; Kayne, Martha; and Mittleider, Kathy. "Putting More Pep in Parenting." *American Journal of Nursing,* Vol. 77 No. 6 (June, 1977), 994-995.

Kalkman, Marian. *Psychiatric Nursing.* McGraw-Hill Book Company: New York, 1967.

Lidz, Theodore. *The Person: His Development Throughout the Life Cycle.* Basic Books, Inc.: New York, 1968.

Maier, Henry, ed. *Three Theories of Child Development.* Harper and Row: New York, 1965.

Murray, Ruth, and Zentner, Judith. *Nursing Assessment and Health Promotion Through the Life Span.* Prentice-Hall, Inc.: Englewood Cliffs, New Jersey, 1975.

Neill, A. S. *Summerhill.* Hart Publishing Company: New York, 1964.

Papalia, Diane E., and Olds, Sally Wendkos. *Human Development.* McGraw-Hill Book Company: New York, 1978.

Pressey, Sidney L., and Kuhlen, Raymond G. *Psychological Development Through the Life Span.* Harper and Row Publishers: New York, 1957.

Richmond, P. G. *An Introduction to Paiget.* Basic Books, Inc.: New York, 1971.

Sarnoff, Charles. *Latency.* Jason Aronson, Inc.: New York, 1976.

Spock, Benjamin. *Baby and Child Care.* Pocket Books: New York, 1976.

Sullivan, Harry Stack. *Personal Psychopathology.* W. W. Norton and Company, Inc.: New York, 1972.

Thompson, Clare. "The Different Schools of Psychoanalysis." *American Journal of Nursing,* Vol. 57 No. 10 (October, 1957), 1304-1307.

chapter 11

the feeling components of personality

learning objectives
On completion of this chapter the reader should be able to:

1 Define *anxiety, conflict, frustration* and *hostility*.
2 Identify the causes of each of these feeling states.
3 Recognize the resultant physiological and psychological effects produced by each of these feelings.

Love, joy, fear and anger are the four basic universal feelings inherent in each person. As the individual progresses through the developmental cycle, he reacts to situations in ways that tend to defend, subdue, change and increase or decrease these basic feeling states. These alterations are a natural and normal part of the developmental process. As the individual progresses toward maturity, he learns how to successfully adapt, adjust or modify his behavior so that emotional equilibrium is maintained. The feeling components of personality which are produced as a result of these alterations are gratification, satisfaction or dissatisfaction in the form of *anxiety, conflict, frustration* or *hostility*.

The nurse's understanding of these feeling components becomes significant as she begins the assessment process. These concepts act as a basis or frame of reference for identifying where the patient is either along the health or illness continuum and from which point intervention may be required to be initiated. The following schematic representations define and illustrate these feeling components of personality as they exist and operate within the individual.

anxiety

Anxiety is a feeling state in which the individual experiences a pervasive, occasionally vague, intense sensation of apprehension or impending disaster. The sensation of anxiety is felt in varying degrees of intensity. Mild anxiety is a necessary and vital component of daily living. Its presence acts as a motivating force toward the problem-solving process. In moderate anxiety more deviant physical, psychological and behavioral changes are noted together with a decreased ability to mobilize defenses to resolve problems and stress. When an individual experiences great anxiety, he loses ability to function, manifests marked physical changes and remains emotionally inert while being overwhelmed with continuous feelings of impending doom. Figure 11-1 outlines the causes that produce the altered feeling state of anxiety and show how the individual responds psychologically and physiologically to the force of anxiety as a mobilizing and/or immobilizing agent.

conflict

Conflict is a feeling state, either conscious or unconscious, in which the individual experiences a clash between two or more equally strong, opposing forces. It engenders confusion around the decision-making process resulting in the individual's inability to make a choice. In conflict an individual may have ambivalent and opposite feelings such as love and hate, trust and distrust. The indecision and ambivalence produce manifest physical and psychological responses. During any period of conflict an individual is often observed to demonstrate two or more of the symptoms illustrated in Figure 11-2.

frustration

Frustration is a feeling state in which the individual experiences interference in the ability to achieve a specific goal, attain satisfaction of a need or solve a problem. The sources of frustration are not the goal, need, or problem *per se*, but rather the barriers encountered by the individual. These barriers may be either internal or external. Internal barriers include the individual's personality characteristics or specific ego strengths and weaknesses; the lack of specific coping abilities; or the inability to manipulate the number of available alterna-

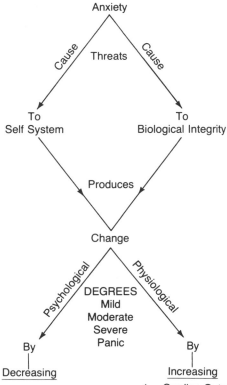

Anxiety

Cause / Threats \ Cause

To
Self System

To
Biological Integrity

Produces

Change

Psychological / DEGREES \ Physiological
Mild
Moderate
Severe
Panic

By
Decreasing

1. Alertness
2. Ability to Perceive
3. Ability to Learn
4. Ability to Receive Sensory Stimuli
5. Ability to Perform
6. Ability to Mobilize Defenses
7. Ability to Communicate
8. Ability to Function Sexually

By
Increasing

1. Cardiac Output
2. Respiratory Rate
3. Adrenalin Flow
4. Muscular Tension
5. Urinary Output
6. Inertia
7. Pain and Agitation
8. Possible Integumentary Breakdown

Figure 11-1

tives. External barriers would include such factors as environmental or situational conditions; overriding authority imposed by others or the exigencies imposed by a specific system of operation. Hence, all people experience "frustrating situations," as a part of daily life. During such situations the individual is generally aware of other feelings within him that are the effect of the frustration. Unlike severe anxiety, frustration allows the individual to

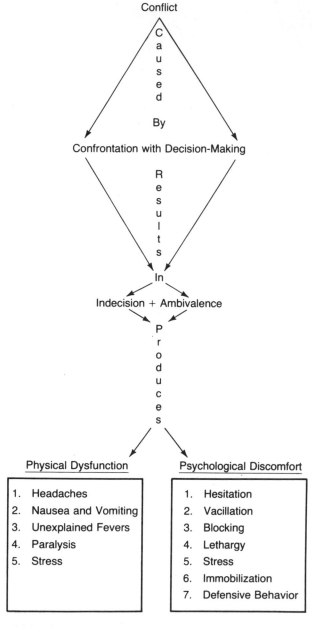

Conflict

Caused

By

Confrontation with Decision-Making

Results

In

Indecision + Ambivalence

Produces

Physical Dysfunction	Psychological Discomfort
1. Headaches	1. Hesitation
2. Nausea and Vomiting	2. Vacillation
3. Unexplained Fevers	3. Blocking
4. Paralysis	4. Lethargy
5. Stress	5. Stress
	6. Immobilization
	7. Defensive Behavior

Figure 11-2

utilize his abilities to select one or more alternative choices of action. In some instances, we see individuals who choose to procrastinate rather than make definitive choices to resolve the sources of frustration. In other instances, we see individuals who respond to frustration by engaging in aggressive acting

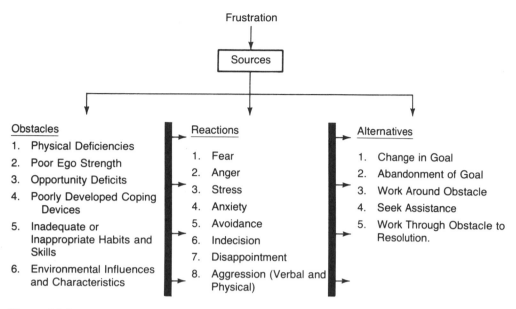

Figure 11-3

out, either verbally or physically. In Figure 11-3, some of the most prevalent and observable results of frustration are outlined.

hostility

Hostility is a feeling state in which the individual, consciously or unconsciously, experiences a sense of helplessness and/or hopelessness with persons or objects and directs negative attitudes or actions toward them. Hostility is the result of repeated frustrations during which the individual experiences intensified feelings of inadequacy, inferiority and the belief that he is being used. Such intensified experiences result in clearly defined acting out as well as in covert signs of negativism. Like anxiety, conflict and frustration, hostility is experienced in varying degrees of intensity and produces a wide range of behaviors. As a feeling state it is one of the most prevalent and diffuse of human emotions. *Overt* hostility is one of the easiest of human emotions to observe, identify and handle with the individual. *Covert* hostility is much less easily discernible since it is masked by apparent friendliness, joviality, and witticisms which tend to make the listener or the recipient uncomfortable without fully realizing the source of the discomfort. Figure 11-4 shows schematically the basic construct of hostility and its effects upon the individual and those around him.

In this chapter we have presented the four major feeling components of personality—anxiety, conflict, frustration and hostility. As illustrated, it becomes clear that these components are an integral part of the developmental process and, therefore, they are feeling states each reader has experienced. In Chapter 16 we will briefly discuss these feelings as they are affected by

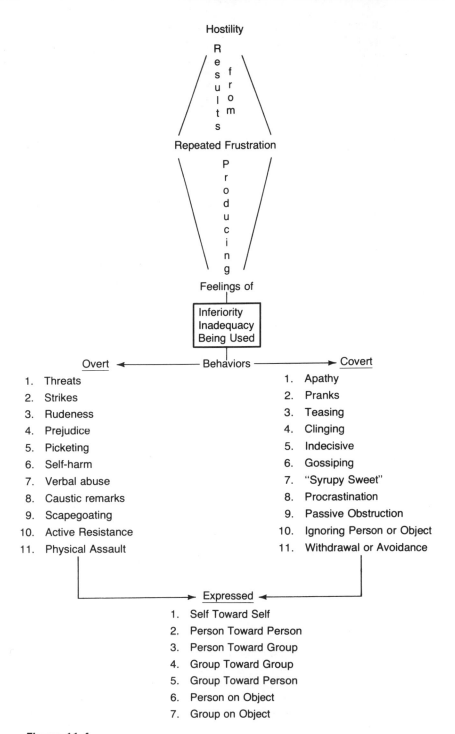

Hostility

R
e   f
s   r
u   o
l   m
t
s

Repeated Frustration

P
r
o
d
u
c
i
n
g

Feelings of

Inferiority
Inadequacy
Being Used

Overt ◄———————— Behaviors ————————► Covert

1. Threats	1. Apathy
2. Strikes	2. Pranks
3. Rudeness	3. Teasing
4. Prejudice	4. Clinging
5. Picketing	5. Indecisive
6. Self-harm	6. Gossiping
7. Verbal abuse	7. "Syrupy Sweet"
8. Caustic remarks	8. Procrastination
9. Scapegoating	9. Passive Obstruction
10. Active Resistance	10. Ignoring Person or Object
11. Physical Assault	11. Withdrawal or Avoidance

Expressed

1. Self Toward Self
2. Person Toward Person
3. Person Toward Group
4. Group Toward Group
5. Group Toward Person
6. Person on Object
7. Group on Object

Figure 11-4

environmental and psychogenic pathology concomitant nursing interventions.

suggested readings

Carter, Frances Monet. *Psychosocial Nursing.* MacMillan Publishing Co., Inc.: New York, 1976.

Coffman, Judith Ann. "Anger: Its Significance for Nurses who Work With Emotionally Disturbed Children." *Perspectives in Psychiatric Care,* Vol. 7, No. 3 (1969), 104-111.

"Dealing with Rage." *Nursing 75,* Vol. 5 No. 10 (October, 1975), 25-29.

Flynn, Gertrude E. "Hostility in a Mad, Mad World." *Perspectives in Psychiatric Care,* Vol. 7 No. 4 (1969), 152-158.

Francis, Gloria M., and Munjas, Barbara. *Promoting Psychological Comfort.* Wm. C. Brown Company: Dubuque, Iowa, 1968.

Frankl, Victor E. *Man's Search for Meaning.* Pocket Books: New York, 1971.

Gruber, Karen A., and Schniewind, Henry E., Jr. "Letting Anger Work for You." *American Journal of Nursing,* Vol. 76 No. 9 (September, 1976), 1450-1452.

Hahn, Jeanette, and Burns, Kenneth R. "Mrs. Richard, A Rabbit and Remotivation." *American Journal of Nursing,* Vol. 73 No. 2 (February, 1973), 302-305.

Kerr, Norine J. "Anxiety: Theoretical Considerations." *Perspectives in Psychiatric Care,* Vol. 16 No. 1 (January-February, 1978), 36-40, 46.

Kimmel, Mary E. "The Age of Anxiety: General Societal Impact and Particular Effects on Criminality." *Journal of Psychiatric Nursing and Mental Health Services,* Vol. 15 No. 11 (November, 1977), 27-30.

Leninger, M. M. "Conflict and Conflict Resolutions: Theories and Processes Relevant to the Health Professions." *American Nurse,* Vol. 6 (December, 1974), 17-22.

Madow, Leo, M.D. *Anger.* Charles Scribner's Sons: New York, 1972.

May, Rollo. *The Meaning of Anxiety.* The Ronald Press: New York, 1950.

McBride, Angela Barron. "The Anger-Depression Guild Go-Round." *American Journal of Nursing,* Vol. 73 No. 6 (June, 1973), 1045-1049.

Moritz, Derry Ann. "Understanding Anger." *American Journal of Nursing,* Vol. 78 No. 1 (January, 1978), 81-83.

Nelson, Priscilla. "Involvement with Betty: An Experience in Reality Therapy." *American Journal of Nursing,* Vol. 74 No. 8 (August, 1974), 1440-1441.

Penalver, Meg. "Helping the Child Handle His Aggression." *American Journal of Nursing,* Vol. 73, No. 9 (September, 1973), 1554-1555.

Penningrath, Philip E. "Control of Violence in a Mental Health Setting." *American Journal of Nursing,* Vol. 75 No. 4 (April, 1975), 606-609.

Peplau, Hildegard E. *Interpersonal Relations in Nursing.* G. P. Putnam's Sons: New York, 1952.

Roche Laboratories. *Aspects of Anxiety.* J. P. Lippincott Co.: Philadelphia, 1965.

Schwartzman, Sylvia T. "Anxiety and Depression in the Stroke Patient: A Nursing Challenge." *Journal of Psychiatric Nursing and Mental Health Services,* Vol. 14 No. 7 (July, 1976), 13-17.

Scott John Paul. *Aggression.* 3d ed. University of Chicago Press: Chicago, Illinois, 1967.

Sobel, David E. "Human Caring." *American Journal of Nursing,* Vol. 69 No. 12 (December, 1969), 2612-2613.

———. "Love and Pain." *American Journal of Nursing,* Vol. 72 No. 5 (May, 1972), 910.

———. "Death and Dying." *American Journal of Nursing,* Vol. 74 No. 1 (January, 1974), 98-99.

———. "Human Violence." *American Journal of Nursing,* Vol. 76 No. 1 (January, 1976), 69-72.

Sullivan, Harry S. *The Psychiatric Interview.* W. W. North & Co.: New York, 1954.

Thomas, Mary D.; Baker, Joan M.; and Estes, Nada J. "Anger: A Tool for Developing Self-Awareness." *American Journal of Nursing,* Vol. 70 No. 12 (December, 1970), 2586-2590.

Veninga, Robert. "Defensive Behavior: Causes, Effects and Cures." *Nursing Digest,* Vol. 3 No. 3 (May/June, 1975), 58-59.

Watson, Jean. "The Quasi-Rational Element in Conflict: A Review of Selected Conflict Literature." *Nursing Research,* Vol. 25 No. 1 (January/February, 1976), 19-23.

Werner, Anita. "The Angry Patient." *Innovations in Nurse-Patient Relationships: Automatic or Reasoned Nurse Actions.* American Nurses Association: New York, 1962, 20-26.

chapter 12

stress and crisis in living: definition and dynamics

learning objectives
On completion of this chapter the reader should be able to:

1 Define *stress, stressor* and *crisis*.
2 Identify the stages of stress.
3 Distinguish between *stress* and *crisis*.
4 Differentiate between *predictable* and *unpredictable crisis*.
5 Understand the part stress and crisis play in the developmental process.

Stress and crisis are phenomena encountered by all living organisms. Therefore, in developing an understanding of people as living, growing, maturing and whole beings, the nurse must know the part these two phenomena play within the total construct of a person's development. The entire process of growth and development is a progressive series of adaptations in which stress plays a significant role. Stress is undue pressure, either real or perceived. It is experienced by individuals within their frame of reference. It is often precipitated by the expectations the individual has for himself and those expectations he believes others have of him. Stress is pressure of varying degrees—pressure to mature, to choose, to learn, to develop skills, to perform, to love, to share, to develop values and to make judgments and decisions. In effect, stress may be described as an automobile an individual maneuvers through his life; the gas pedal and the brake are analogous to the individual's coping devices. The amount of perceived or real pressure causes the individual to manipulate the gas pedal and the brake. The degree to which the individual allows the automobile to get out of his control is the difference between function and dysfunction. Stress is a normal, recurring event inherent in daily living and so cannot be avoided.

Stress is created or enhanced by a stressor. *A stressor* is any agent, condition, situation, goal, feeling, thought or behavior which demands an increase in any vital activity within the autonomic or central nervous system of the individual. The stress syndrome or general adaptive syndrome, as it is sometimes called, is divided into three stages: 1) the stage of alarm reaction in which the individual mobilizes defensive forces; 2) the stage of resistance which reflects the individual's use of the full adaptive response pattern to the stressor; and 3) the stage of exhaustion which reflects the individual's need for rest and recuperation.

Stress produces change. The change may be either physiological or psychological, either healthy and useful or unhealthy and destructive to the individual. The destructive results of the stress may be irreversible, depending on the degree of damage sustained by the individual. Stress can be monitored, quantified and analyzed at any point through the assessment of an individual's responsive behavior.

Mild stress is an integral part of the developmental process. It can clearly be seen in the cyclical pattern manifested in the growth and development of every child. For example, in the two-year-old stress is intense due to the stressors of rapid physical growth and the insatiable desire to discover the self and the environment. The result is the "Terrible Two" who is active, energetic, apparently purposeless, easily distracted—a curious and complex organism who strives to do everything and is continuously in motion. The three-year-old, on the other hand, experiences less stress as he gains confidence in his ability to handle himself and his environment. Thus, the "Trusting Three" has slowed down and begins to assimilate, integrate and refine previous learning. The cycle continues with periods of heightened growth and activity followed by periods of rest and integration. This pattern becomes visible at birth, continues throughout one's life span and terminates only by death.

Crisis is a form of severe stress. It differs from stress in that crisis is time-limited and is usually precipitated by new or sudden situations or forces. Crisis leaves the individual with an overwhelming feeling of devastation and futility so that preexistant adaptive, alternative, resolving or coping mechanisms are ineffectual. During crisis or continued undue stress the individual frequently loses his ability to mobilize his capacity to resolve problems and seek alternative measures. This immobilization can be a temporary loss or a more pronounced dysfunction lasting the duration of the crisis. There are crises in every life, and they occur at all ages. Some individuals experience more crises than others; some are better able to cope with crises than others.

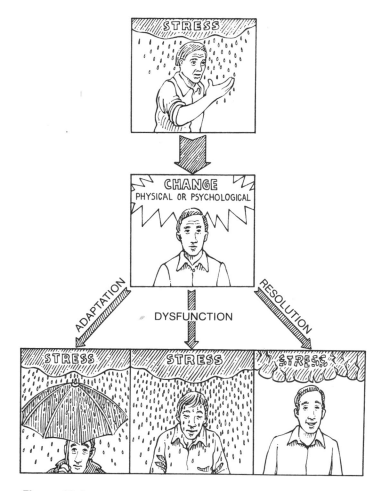

Figure 12-1

Therefore, it can be said that some types of crises are universal; they occur in the lives of all persons and are thereby predictable. However, most crises are unpredictable and hence, are unique to the individual. Some examples of predictable crises in the daily living experience of an individual are the moment of birth, the first date, marriage and retirement. Some situations which might occur in the individual's life experience and be viewed as unpredictable are sudden illness, loss of a job, loss of a loved one, separation or divorce, or severe financial reverses.

These stressors can be intrinsic, that is, occurring within the individual; extrinsic, meaning arising from persons, places and situations around the individual or, more commonly, a combination of both factors. Notwithstanding

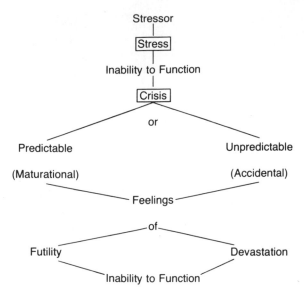

Figure 12-2

its sources, crisis is an intense physical and emotionally demanding period of time for the individual.

In Figure 12-2 the progression of stress and its effects from the onset to the point of "inability to function" is traced. It is generally at this point that the patient is amenable to intervention, comes to seek help and is sometimes hospitalized for treatment. It is essential that the nurse understand this concept so that she can maximize the use of communication and the therapeutic self on behalf of the patient's well-being.

suggested readings

Aguilera, D. C., and Messick, J. M. *Crisis Intervention: Theory and Methodology.* C. V. Mosby Company: St. Louis, 1974.

Benson, Herbert. "Your Innate Asset for Combating Stress." *Nursing Digest,* Vol. 3 No. 3 (May/June 1975), 38-41.

Carter, Frances Monet. *Psychosocial Nursing.* 2d ed. MacMillan Publishing, Inc.: New York, 1976.

Clark, Terri Patrice. "Counseling Victims of Rape." *American Journal of Nursing,* Vol. 76 No. 12 (December 1976), 1964-1966.

Dohrenwend, Barbara Snell, and Dohrenwend, Bruce P., eds. *Stressful Life Events: Their Nature and Effects.* John Wiley & Sons: New York, 1974.

Ewing, Charles P. *Crisis Intervention as Psychotherapy.* Oxford University Press, New York: 1978.

Graber, Richard F. "When Divorce Crisis is the Diagnosis." *Patient Care: The Journal of Practical Family Medicine,* Vol. XI No. 6 (March 15, 1977), 90-91, 95-123.

Hitchcock, Janice Marland. "Crisis Intervention—The Pebble in the Pool." *American Journal of Nursing,* Vol. 73 No. 8 (August, 1973), 1388-1390.

King, Joan. "The Initial Interview: Basis for Assessment in Crisis Intervention." *Perspectives in Psychiatric Care,* Vol. 9 No. 6 (1971), 247-256.

Maloney, Elizabeth. "The Subjective and Objective Definition of Crisis." *Perspectives in Psychiatric Care,* Vol. 9 No. 6 (1971), 257-268.

Marcinck, Margaret Boyle. "Stress in the Surgical Patient." *American Journal of Nursing,* Vol. 77 No. 11 (November 1977), 1809-1811.

Messick, Janice. "Crisis Intervention Concepts: Implications for Nursing Practices." *Journal of Psychiatric and Mental Health Services,* Vol. 10 No. 5 (1972), 3-5.

Miller, Catherine M. "Crisis Intervention and Health Counseling: An Overview." *School Health Review* (September, 1970), 16-17.

Parad, Howard J., ed. *Crisis Intervention: Selected Readings.* Family Service Association of America: New York, 1965.

Reichle, Marian J. "Psychological Stress in The Intensive Care Unit." *Nursing Digest,* Vol. 3 No. 3 (May/June 1975), 12-15.

Saranson, Irwin G., and Spielberger, Charles D. *Stress and Anxiety.* Vols. I and II. Hemisphere Publishing Corp.: Washington D.C. 1975.

Selye, Hans. *The Stress of Life.* McGraw-Hill Book Company: New York, 1956.

———. "The Stress Syndrome." *American Journal of Nursing,* Vol. 65 No. 3 (March, 1965), 97-99.

Stephenson, Carol A. "Stress in Critically Ill Patients." *American Journal of Nursing,* Vol. 77 No. 11, (November, 1977) 1806-1809.

Stubbs, Diane Cronin. "Family Crisis. Intervention: A study." *Journal of Psychiatric Nursing and Mental Health Services,* Vol. 16 No. 1 (January, 1978), 36-44.

chapter 13

mental mechanisms:
automatic coping devices

learning objectives
On completion of this chapter the reader should be able to:

1 Define the term *mental mechanisms*.
2 Explain how mental mechanisms are used.
3 List the purpose and function of each mechanism.
4 Identify and differentiate between each of the mental mechanisms cited.

Mental mechanisms are intrapsychic devices, ego defenses. They are adjustment techniques which serve as a constructive means for the maintenance of emotional equilibrum and, as such, are used by all people in their day-to-day lives. Through observation of behavior, the nurse becomes aware of the existence and the manner in which these mechanisms operate within an individual.

Mental mechanisms are those specific defensive operations existing outside of and beyond conscious awareness. The primary functions of the mechanisms are to facilitate the resolution of emotional conflict; provide relief from stress; cushion emotional pain, and to avoid or alleviate anxiety. In essence, they serve to protect and maintain the individual's self-esteem and ego identity from the continuous blows of reality. Excessive reliance on and inappropriate use of these mechanisms may lead to the development of pathological symptomatology within the individual.

TABLE 13-1
THE DEFENSE MECHANISMS

Mechanism	Definition	Interpretation	Examples
1) Compensation	A mechanism by which the individual seeks to make up for or offset deficiencies, either real or imagined.	It is a disguising mechanism and involves an attempt to meet self-imposed standards thereby preserving self-respect. It is a means of overcoming failure or frustration in some sphere of activity by overemphasizing another.	An undersized young man becomes a bantamweight prizefighter. An unattractive and unpopular girl cultivates intellectual abilities and is on the honor roll at school.
2) Conversion	A mechanism through which elements of intrapsychic conflict are disguised and expressed symbolically through physical symptoms.	Used to rechannel and externalize unbearable feelings.	A young mother, when told she was going to have twins, becomes blind. Mr. Jones develops laryngitis the evening before he is scheduled to give a speech at a business lunch.
3) Denial	A mechanism by which the ego refuses to perceive or face emotional conflict.	It is an escape mechanism which allows the individual to move away from the unpleasant reality as if it did not exist.	A patient with a cerebral vascular accident refuses to attend physical therapy, saying, "There's nothing wrong, all I need is rest." A comment often heard from patients in a psychiatric unit: "I have no problem, I don't need to talk with you."
4) Displacement	A mechanism through which emotional feeling is transferred, deflected and redirected from one idea, person or object to another.	It is a disguising mechanism which uses a convenient, less threatening target to release emotional drives.	The boss berates Mr. Smith for a mistake. That evening Mr. Smith yells at his wife because dinner is ten minutes late.

152

TABLE 13-1 (continued)

Mechanism	Definition	Interpretation	Examples
4) Displacement (continued)			Jane does not make the cheer-leading team at school, and when she comes home tears down all the football posters in her room.
5) Disassociation	A mechanism through which the effective emotional significance is separated and detached from an idea, situation, object or relationship.	Its use allows the individual to isolate or compartmentalize painful feelings.	Jim grins and smiles as he relates the details about his automobile accident. Some clinical examples include somnambulism (sleep walking), traumatic amnesia or fugue states.
6) Identification	A mechanism by which an individual patterns himself to resemble the personality and traits of an admired other.	It is a disguising mechanism used as an attempt to preserve the ego ideal. Its use contributes to ego development but does not replace the person's own ego. Not exclusively linked with a decrease in anxiety.	An adolescent girl adopts the mannerisms and style of dress of a particular recording star. A young man chooses to become a draftsman just like his father.
7) Introjection	A mechanism through which loved or hated attitudes, wishes, ideals, values, objects or persons are symbolically incorporated into self.	It is a denying and disguising mechanism in which the ego structure is changed to keep the individual free from threat.	While playing, 5-year-old Tommy says to his pal Joey, "Don't get dirty, it's not nice." The patient who claims to be Jesus Christ.
8) Projection	A mechanism through which the individual rejects aspects of self by imputing to others motives and emotional feelings which are unacceptable to self.	It is a refusal to acknowledge undesirable or instinctual impulses in order to protect the self.	Archie Bunker calls Edith a "ding bat." A secretary says, "All the girls in the office are jealous of my position and want to take over my job."

TABLE 13-1 (continued)

Mechanism	Definition	Interpretation	Examples
9) Rationalization	A mechanism through which the ego justifies or attempts to modify otherwise unacceptable impulses, needs, feelings, behavior, and motives into ones which are consciously tolerable and acceptable.	It is a disguising and self-deceptive mechanism used to increase self-esteem and to obtain and retain social approval and acceptance.	Mrs. Ferris, who can't afford to buy a new dress, says to her friend Stella, "I'd love to have the dress in that window but I don't think the color suits me." While at a party, Mr. Peters says, "I'll have one more drink. I don't have far to go."
10) Reaction Formation	A mechanism through which an individual assumes attitudes, motives, or needs which are opposite to consciously disowned ones.	It is a protective drive which serves to prevent the emergence of painful, undesirable and unacceptable attitudes.	A young mother who is unaware of her hostile feelings toward her child becomes overprotective toward the child. Mr. Brown is extremely polite and courteous toward his mother-in-law, whom he intensely dislikes.
11) Regression	A mechanism through which an individual retreats to an earlier and subjectively more comfortable level of adjustment.	It is a denying and protective mechanism which allows the individual to retreat from reality, reduce anxiety and become more dependent.	A 4-year-old begins to suck his thumb and wet the bed shortly after the birth of a sibling. Doris, 18, flies into a temper tantrum when she can't have her own way.
12) Repression	A mechanism in which there is automatic and involuntary submerging of unpleasant or painful thoughts, feelings and impulses into the unconscious.	It is the primary forgetting and protective mechanism used by the ego. All other mechanisms reinforce it. Repressed material is not subject to conscious recall.	Mr. Willis can't remember attempting to commit suicide. Mary, an unmarried, pregnant 20 year old, can't remember the name of the baby's father.

TABLE 13-1 (continued)

Mechanism	Definition	Interpretation	Examples
13) *Sublimation*	A mechanism through which instinctual drives which are consciously intolerable, or which are blocked and unattainable, are then directed into channels that are personally and socially acceptable.	It is the most efficient and creative of the defense mechanisms and serves to channel libidinal energy into constructive activities.	A man who has strong competitive or aggressive drives channels his energy into building up a successful business. A young unmarried woman derives satisfaction from taking care of neighborhood children.
14) *Substitution*	A mechanism through which a goal, emotion, drive, attitude or need which is consciously unacceptable is replaced by one that is more acceptable.	It is a disguising mechanism used to reduce frustration and promote satisfaction.	A rejected boy friend "rushes" into marriage on the rebound. The dependence on the use of alcohol or drugs.
15) *Suppression*	A mechanism in which there is a deliberate, intentional exclusion of thoughts, feelings or experiences from the conscious mind.	It is a voluntary forgetting and postponing mechanism used to preserve the status quo and protect self-esteem.	Mr. Gordon carries the bills in his pocket before remembering to mail in the payments. During finals week, Lucy says, "I'll watch just one T.V. program before I study."
16) *Symbolization*	A mechanism through which an external object becomes an outward representation of an internal idea, wish, attitude or feeling.	It is a disguising, compensatory mechanism which is used as a vehicle for emotional self-expression.	Carey remarked to her friend, "you have a heart of gold." A boy sends his girl friend a dozen red roses.
17) *Undoing*	A mechanism through which an individual endeavors to actually or symbolically erase a previous consciously intolerable action or experience.	It is a disguising and restoring mechanism to alleviate guilt and anxiety.	A mother who has just punished her child decides to bake cookies. A religious, single girl who engages in sexual activity with her boy friend goes to church and lights candles.

In Table 13-1, we identify, define, interpret and provide examples for some of the more common ego defenses. In studying this chart, the nurse will note that the defense mechanisms tend to overlap and that there is a close interrelationship between the mechanisms particularly with regard to purpose and function. The examples used to illustrate each of the mechanisms point out specific instances in which these mechanisms become operational. However, the nurse must keep in mind that in a reality situation, mental mechanisms seldom operate in total isolation, one from another, but rather, they tend to be used in combination.

Observation and scrutiny of the mental mechanisms make them real for us. Not surprisingly, we can identify parts of ourselves as we read the examples. Mental mechanisms are the fiber of daily functioning which we use to handle stress, crisis, human emotions and to assist us in fostering maturation and growth. These mechanisms are vitally important to understand as a part of our own daily patterns of behavior so that we can then develop a more perceptive therapeutic self. Their presentation in this outline form is an effort to stress their importance and give the reader an easy, accessible reference to use in nursing practice.

suggested readings

Bell, Janice M. "Stressful Life Events and Coping Methods in Mental-Illness and Wellness Behaviors." *Nursing Research,* Vol. 26, No. 2 (March/April, 1977), 136-140.

English, Spurgeon O., and Pearson, T. H. J. *Emotional Problems of Living,* 3d ed. W. W. Norton and Co., Inc.: New York, 1963.

Freud, Anna. *The Ego and Mechanisms of Defense.* International Universities Press: New York, 1946.

Laughlin, H. *The Ego and Its Defenses.* Appleton-Century Crofts: New York, 1970.

chapter 14

psychopathology: symptoms, dynamics, and principles

learning objectives

On completion of this chapter, the reader should be able to:

1 Define *psychopathology*.
2 Identify, define and describe the most commonly encountered and treated psychiatric disorders.
3 Explain the differences in etiology of the five major categories of psychopathology.
4 Identify the characteristic symptomotology associated with the five major categories.
5 Explain the dynamics associated with the five categories.
6 Identify the general concepts and principles which are specifically related to each of the diagnostic categories.
7 Integrate and apply the general concepts and principles in the development of written nursing care plans for individual patients.

psychopathology: an overview

Psychopathology is a term used to designate the study of disease processes of the mind: the persistent, recognizable and exaggerated expressions of thinking, feeling and behaving. Psychopathology encompasses the causes, symptomatic manifestations and dynamics affecting the mind and thereby the individual's total pattern of action and reaction in his daily life. This chapter presents an overview and synthesis of five major commonly encountered syndromes: 1) psychoneuroses, 2) psychophysiological autonomic and visceral disorders, 3) personality disorders, 4) psychoses and 5) acute and chronic brain syndromes. This chapter is by no means meant to be a comprehensive survey of psychiatric disorders. There are many available resources in both books and journals to which the reader may refer for detailed descriptions, as well as particulars of nomenclature and treatment. This chapter is designed to be of practical value and is limited to essential information. There is no special association or adherence to any one particular theoretical school of thought. It is a composite summation of data and nomenclature regarding specific disease conditions, their distinguishing characteristics, etiology, dynamics and the major concepts and principles underlying nursing care.

To orient the reader to the complexity of psychopathology and to provide an essential frame of reference, the chart below outlines each of the five major syndromes. The reader will note that each of the broad classifications have certain dynamics or underlying causes in common, such as some form of subjective distress; exaggerated or excessive reliance on the automatic adaptive mechanisms; disturbed interpersonal relationships; ineffective communication; inability to delay gratification; and an inability to meet and satisfy wants, needs or desires in one or more areas of vital functioning. Nevertheless, each of the five major syndromes are diagnostically and therapeutically different. Specifically, they differ in definition, specific types, etiology, characteristics, distinctive dynamics and broad general concepts and principles on which nursing intervention is based.

Table 14-1 provides an outlined, concise synthesis of commonly encountered and treated psychopathologies. We highlighted many fundamental theoretical and technical concepts in a condensed, readily comprehensible format which is intended to assist the reader to become better able to identify the major categories and also to more easily identify the etiology, dynamics and characteristics manifested by individuals suffering from these types of mental disorders. In order to better assist with the integration of theory and practice, the last segment of the outilne is devoted to expounding a few of the more pronounced concepts and principles for nursing care and intervention. In other chapters of this book the reader will find extensive and detailed descriptions of theory and practice principles of therapeutic interventions relating to stress and crisis, human feelings, depression, communicative skills and the therapeutic use of self. Careful reading and review of the significant chapters arm the reader with those essential skills necessary to effectively intervene and therapeutically advocate for those patients suffering the ravages of psychopathology and to plan for effective and fecund nursing care.

In the subsequent pages we have elaborated on the five major categories of psychopathology so that the reader may learn to identify the characteristic symptomotology associated with each of the disorders.

TABLE 14-1
DESCRIPTIVE ANALYSIS OF DISEASE CONDITIONS

	Psychoneurosis	Psychophysiologic Autonomic and Visceral Disorders (Psychosomatic)	Personality Disorders	Psychosis	Acute and Chronic Brain Disorders
Definition	A psychological disability resulting from an individual's inability to cope with emotional conflicts or stressful environmental problems.	A maladaptive emotional reaction in which the symptoms are expressed in organs innervated by the autonomic nervous system producing physiologic change concurrent with psychological disequilibrium.	Entrenched, chronic, maladaptive characterologic patterns in which an individual experiences little or no anxiety or guilt.	Psychogenic reactions in which the individual experiences severe personality disorganization and disintegration along with marked distortions of reality.	A disorder in which the individual sustains psychological and physiological dysfunction as a consequence of damaged brain tissue.
Types	Anxiety neurosis Phobic neurosis Conversion neurosis Dissociative neurosis Depressive neurosis Obsessive-compulsive neurosis	Gastrointestinal reactions a) Peptic ulcer b) Ulcerative colitis Cardiovascular reactions a) Essential hypertension b) Migraine Respiratory reactions a) Bronchial asthma b) Hyperventilation syndrome	Personality disorders a) Schizoid b) Paranoid c) Inadequate d) Passive-aggressive e) Antisocial Sexual deviation Alcoholism Drug dependence Maladjustment reactions to living	Schizophrenia a) Simple b) Hebephrenic c) Catatonic d) Paranoid e) Schizoaffective f) Chronic undifferentiated g) Childhood schizophrenia Major affective disorders a) Manic-depressive: manic	Delirium tremens Korsakoff's syndrome Cerebral arteriosclerosis Intercranial neoplasms Brain trauma Encephalitis Systemic intoxication or poisioning and others

TABLE 14-1 (continued)

	Psychoneurosis	Psychophysiologic Autonomic and Visceral Disorders (Psychosomatic)	Personality Disorders	Psychosis	Acute and Chronic Brain Disorders
Types (continued)		Genitourinary reactions a) Impotence or frigidity b) Amenorrhea Musculoskeletal reactions a) Functional backache b) Rheumatoid arthritis Skin reactions a) Psoriasis b) Neurodermatitis Endocrine reactions a) Diabetes mellitus b) Hyperthyroidism		b) Manic-depressive: depressed Involutional melancholia Paranoid states	
Etiology	Disruption in the developmental pattern or in interpersonal experiences. Multiple, intrapsychic conflicts resulting from unresolved guilt, fear, prolonged stress or crisis.	Internalization of feelings. Internalization of negative emotions. Internal discharge of negative emotions. Constitutional organ susceptibility.	Faulty or arrested emotional development which interferes with adequate social control or superego formation. Constitutional predisposition. Deprivation of basic	Multiple causality, most likely a combination of biochemical, social, and psychological factors.	Any condition or agent which produces central nervous system pathology and cerebral tissue impairment.

TABLE 14-1 (continued)

	Psychoneurosis	Psychophysiologic Autonomic and Visceral Disorders (Psychosomatic)	Personality Disorders	Psychosis	Acute and Chronic Brain Disorders
Etiology (continued)	Conflict between what patient believes society expects and the bi-personal self. Underlying and sustained conflict arising from the dichotomy of bicultures and subcultures.		needs in early childhood. Physical and/or emotional trauma in childhood or adolescence.		
Characteristics	A strong sense of personal discomfort; heightened levels of anxiety. Major personality organization remains intact. Maintains contact with reality. Maintains usual roles, activities or employment. Decreased productivity and creativity. Fixed attitudes, affections and/or mannerisms.	Organ pathology. Physical illness is the expression of prolonged or intense emotional stress. Physical rather than emotional symptoms dominate the clinical picture. Excellent ability to overtly mask stress and conflict. If unchecked and unresolved, physical symptoms may be fatal.	Lifelong, repetitive, maladaptive and often self-defeating behavior. Anxiety is not apparent. Seldom seeks help on own initiative. Tolerance to frustration and stress is low. Occasional intellectual insight. Pathology is directed outward toward and against others.	Major personality disorganization. Marked interference with ability to function, personally and interpersonally. Significant discrepancies between thoughts, feelings and behavior. Substitution of fantasy for reality. Presence of delusional and hallucinatory systems. Disorientation in the three spheres.	Reversible or irreversible. Deficits in intellectual functioning. Impaired orientation. Liability of affect. Primary and secondary personality changes. Alterations in the levels of consciousness. Memory and/or speech impairment.

TABLE 14-1 (continued)

	Psychoneurosis	Psychophysiologic Autonomic and Visceral Disorders (Psychosomatic)	Personality Disorders	Psychosis	Acute and Chronic Brain Disorders
Characteristics (continued)	Excessive dependency or domination. Correlation between thought and feeling content.		Frequent confrontation with society's mores, norms and laws.	Regression.	
Dynamics	Unresolved emotional conflict is complicated with underlying feelings of guilt resulting in overwhelming anxiety. Unsatisfactory relationships with parents, siblings or peers in the developmental process. The resultant symptomotology offers the individual an external means of expressing repressed material thereby allowing both primary and secondary gains for the ego.	Psychological stress is converted into anxiety which is directed internally through the autonomic nervous system. The individual experiences pathophysiological functional or structural changes of the organs. Sustained or prolonged conflict causes internalization of fear, hostility and/or guilt.	The individual operates from an egocentric viewpoint and remains narcissistic. Interpersonal relationships are not important unless they can be used to achieve specific need gratification. A concealed "taking" relationship predominates as opposed to a mutual "give and take" relationship. Avoidance of expectations, discomfort and/or stress producing situations.	Loss of ego boundaries. Denial of reality. Severe regression. Security and identity are threatened. Interpersonal relationships are superficial. Failure or inability to trust self or others.	Interference with or destruction of cerebral tissue. Libidinal energy is released as a result of organic changes. Loss of ability to control libidinal drives. Interruption of learning and coping potential.

TABLE 14-1 (continued)

	Psychoneurosis	Psychophysiologic Autonomic and Visceral Disorders (Psychosomatic)	Personality Disorders	Psychosis	Acute and Chronic Brain Disorders
Dynamics (continued)			Disproportionate projection and accusations toward persons, places and objects in the environment.		
Concepts and Principles for Nursing Care	The presence of anxiety is a universal phenomenon. Knowledge and understanding of "normal anxiety" will provide the nurse with a base to assess the level of patient dysfunction. The symptom picture is usually indicative of the underlying conflict. Rituals are accompanied by profound dread and apprehension. All behavior is meaningful. Nursing care is directed toward the re-	Any attitude, behavior or situation which produces a sense of insecurity arouses anxiety. The overt expression of feelings alleviates internal stress. Disturbed family relationships play an important role in the development and outcome of the patient's illness. In psychosomatic illness inter-personal factors and physical disease are woven together in a single process. Effective treatment depends on a dual	A firm, calm, consistent, quiet approach is most effective and will produce the least amount of manipulative or explosive response behavior. The nurse must protect other patients from being manipulated or exploited by an individual with a personality disorder. Give clear, concise explanations and directions to avoid verbal entanglements with the patient. Uniform scheduling and consistent application of firm limit setting offers positive	The attitude of personnel makes or breaks the possibility of recovery for the psychotic patient. Care must be directed toward the maintenance of reality relationships. Genuine interest, honesty, warmth and optimism are essential for establishing contact with psychotic persons. Physical and psychological needs merit equal attention. Familiar routines and persons contribute to security. As a social being,	Cerebral damage produces physiological and psychological malfunctioning. Organic conditions produce mental dysfunction, alteration in mood, physical manifestations and disrupted interpersonal relationships. Acute conditions require immediate interventive techniques to maintain life. Chronic conditions require supportive care coupled with an attitudinal approach of hopefulness. Patients with impaired judgment are

TABLE 14-1 (continued)

	Psychoneurosis	Psychophysiologic Autonomic and Visceral Disorders (Psychosomatic)	Personality Disorders	Psychosis	Acute and Chronic Brain Disorders
Concepts and Principles for Nursing Care (continued)	lief of physical and psychological symptoms. The patient's self-esteem is enhanced by the nurse's demonstration of acceptance, respect and concern for his well-being. Positive, satisfying experiences are introduced to correct developmental and maturational deficits.	emphasis, physical and psychological. A planned schedule of social and recreational activities provides release from tension. Diversion deflects mental preoccupation with self and disability. Know the source or cause of the stresses, tensions or problems creating the physical reactions. Give priority to the exploration of the primary causes of repressed feelings with the patient.	guidance toward establishing self-control. Consistency in decision making enables the nurse to maintain an objective viewpoint.	man's psychological equilibrium needs to be maintained through satisfying relationships with others, both individually and in groups.	unable to function independently and therefore require close observation and protective supervision. Familiarity with the environment promotes feelings of security while change produces frustration. Loss or impairment of physical functioning contributes to increasing the level of fear, anxiety and confusion.

psychoneuroses

The psychoneurotic conditions demonstrate a broad range of responses to overwhelming anxiety. The predominant behavioral pattern within this clinical syndrome is that of ritualism. The clinical symptoms seen within this diagnostic category are viewed as ineffective substitutes for satisfactory need gratification. They are generally of a symbolic nature reflecting the underlying conflict and usually interfere with the maintenance of interpersonal relationships. The underlying conflict can be traced to disturbances within childhood developmental experiences, particularly those in which primal cravings and vital sitmuli were not met or were thwarted and resulted in the imposition of rigid restrictions. In adult life the outcome is conflict which produces tension and the need for defensive and security operations. Thus, the neurotic patient is responding to internal or external stress. His response permits him to avoid the initial stressful situation while allowing him to obtain gratification for his previously unmet dependency needs. The following excerpt from a case history illustrates a rather classical picture of an anxiety neurosis.

> Mr. Starre is a 42-year-old Caucasian married man who works as a foreman in a steel mill. He is the father of three children, two boys and a girl, ages 17, 15 and 12 respectively. In the past two years, he has experienced progressive feelings of acute uneasiness. Originally, he displayed periodic restlessness and evidenced some minor disturbances in his sleep pattern. Gradually, he began to complain of indigestion, palpitations, loss of appetite, constipation, cold sweats, insomnia and impotence. In addition, he became more irritable, short-tempered and demanding, and imposed more and more rigid restrictions, not only on his two sons but also on the men he supervised at work. His sick days began to outnumber his work days. He sought frequent medical assistance but stated that he didn't feel any better despite the variety of medications he was taking. Mr. Starre had been admitted to various hospitals for complete physical examinations and diagnostic evaluation. He refused to believe that all the test results were negative and maintained that he was a "sick man." On his last admission he became very angry when the phsyician suggested that a psychiatric consult should be considered. He demanded that he be discharged so that he could "find himself a doctor who really knows what he was doing."

Mr. Starre's behavior represents a deep-seated and long-term problem. The anxiety displayed has intensified over time so that his total functioning as an individual—as a father, husband and foreman have been severely disrupted. He manifests excessive use of rationalization and denial. If left untreated, more severe ego dysfunction can be anticipated which, in turn, can lead to a complete alienation of his family, friends, and co-workers.

Most authorities believe that psychoneurotic conditions are less severe and disabling than other psychiatric disorders; nevertheless, they can and do produce marked interference with effective and efficient functioning. Table 14-2 outlines in greater detail the chief clinical entities within this broad diagnostic classification and highlights the dynamics, the defensive operations, and the specific symptomotology displayed along with the general concepts and principles for nursing care.

TABLE 14-2
AN OVERVIEW OF PSYCHONEUROTIC REACTIONS

Condition	Definition	Dynamics	Symptom Picture	Concepts and Principles for Nursing Care
1) Anxiety neurosis	A reaction in response to no apparent or insufficient environmental stimulus.	Persistent overuse of *repression* to control emotionally charged thoughts and feelings. The presence of socially unacceptable thoughts, feelings, wants or desires that if actualized would cause loss of approval, acceptance or love from others. Fear of censure, disapproval or rejection threatens the self-concept.	Free floating and recurrent acute anxiety. Dramatic increase in the level and diffusion of anxiety. Somatic symptoms are associated with the autonomic nervous system. Decreased ability to focus on the situation at hand. Interruption of judgment. Sudden onset of panic.	Intervention is imperative before anxiety mounts and becomes uncontrollable. Remaining with the patient and providing a warm, concerned human environment enhances the patient's security and reduces the level of anxiety. The nurse listens carefully to the expression of somatic concerns and does not challenge or cast doubt on their validity.
2) Phobic neurosis	A reaction of intense recurrent, unreasonable fear attached to a specific object or situation.	Incomplete repression wtih *displacement* of anxiety onto an external focus which the individual can then avoid. Particular phobias assume a *symbolic* significance with respect to underlying emotional conflicts or unacceptable desires.	Intense, prolonged irrational and disabling fear. Common phobias include fear of the dark; open and closed spaces; heights; animals and birds; and dirt or germs. Avoidance of socializing behavior and frequent reclusiveness results in eccentricities.	Phobias are *real* to the individual. The nurse demonstrates acceptance of the patient's avoidance patterns as being necessary for his survival. The nurse assumes initiative in seeking out the patient and provides opportunities for the verbal expression of feelings.

TABLE 14-2 (continued)

Condition	Definition	Dynamics	Symptom Picture	Concepts and Principles for Nursing Care
2) Phobic neurosis (continued)				Assisting the patient in exploring the "source" or primary painful life experience or trauma that eventuated in displacement.
3) Conversion neurosis	A reaction in which the individual unconsciously transforms his underlying conflict into specific kinds of motor or sensory dysfunction.	*Conversion* of anxiety into somatic symptoms, *symbolic* of the underlying conflict. Primary gain is relief from emotional tension. Secondary gain is the advantage the symptom provides in meeting the need for dependency. Outcome is the avoidance of responsible, independent functioning. Avoidance of an anticipated, emotionally and/or physically painful experience. *Denial* of an unpleasant and/or uncomfortable reality in one's life.	Physical manifestations in the form of blindness, deafness, aphonia, laryngitis and convulsions. Displays a lack of concern or indifference toward the existing symptom. Minimal observable anxiety.	The individual does not consciously invent or choose the condition. Conversion involves the voluntary and sensory systems. The physical symptoms serve to lessen any consciously felt anxiety. Nursing care is focused on the individual and his feelings, not on his symptoms.

TABLE 14-2 (continued)

Condition	Definition	Dynamics	Symptom Picture	Concepts and Principles for Nursing Care
4) Dissociative neurosis	A reaction in which certain aspects of the individual's personality are split off, separated or detached from his conscious awareness.	Employs mechanisms of *dissociation, conversion* and *symbolism.* Ego attempts to protect itself from critical and/or dangerous pain. *Denial* is used to escape from reality.	Alterations in the state of consciousness, in the person's identity or memory. Depersonalization. Overwhelming anxiety. Manifested through amnesia, fugues and twilight states.	The nurse must view the patient's emotional functioning as the outcome of his growth and developmental process. It is necessary for the nurse to understand the patient's feelings and behavior and not pass judgment on his actions. Understand the dynamics of this problem to maximize interventive techniques.
5) Obsessive-compulsive neurosis	A reaction in which the individual experiences persistent, distressing thoughts or impulses resulting in irresistible acting out behavior.	Unsuccessful repression is reinforced through the use of such defensive responses as: *displacement, reaction formation, undoing and symbolism.*	Ambivalence. Doubt. Vacillation. Persistent, recurring ideation. Repetitive, stereotyped, motor activity.	The patient recognizes the unreasonableness of his obsessions and compulsions. Rituals release tension, and temporarily reduce the level of anxiety. Interruption of ritualistic behavior increases the patient's anxiety and guilt. Protect patient from ridicule. Assist the patient to develop new interests outside self.

TABLE 14-2 (continued)

Condition	Definition	Dynamics	Symptom Picture	Concepts and Principles for Nursing Care
6) Depressive neurosis	A reaction in which the individual experiences a state of sadness due to disappointment, an upsetting life event or a loss of a significant person, possession or position.	Damage to self-esteem with associated repressed anger. Disparity between the superego value system and the ego activity which results in guilt. Feelings of inadequacy and inferiority are more pronounced due to exaggerated ego ideal. Depressive features existent throughout the life experience.	Marked ambivalence. Diffused anger and hostility. Fluctuations in mood. Difficulty in concentration. Reduction in psychomotor activity. Reality oriented. Appetite and sleep disturbances. Somatic complaints. Pessimism. Vacillation between ability to function and immobility. Numerous suicidal threats. Accidental death.	Provide external structure and milieu that gradually allows the patient to assume responsibility for his life experiences. Verbal or behavioral expression of anger or hostility provides a release for internalized emotion. Persuasion is a useful tool for meeting the needs for acceptance and attention. Reassurance is conveyed through the setting of realistic limits. Feelings of adequacy can be promoted by opportunities for achieving small goals. Allow patient to experience success and accomplishment via a short term project.

There are important points for the nurse to remember while caring for the neurotic patient. First, realize that the individual is experiencing *real* discomfort and distress. Second, the overwhelming anxiety and corresponding fears that are felt by the patient are as significant as any physical pain or condition. Third, neurotic symptoms are *consciously* unwanted and viewed by the individual as undesirable; they produce irritation and create distress, are felt to be strange and to produce discontent in daily living. Fourth, the clinical picture is not always definitive and more than one condition or type may exist simultaneously. And fifth, the specific symptoms associated with this diagnostic category are not limited to the psychoneuroses but may also exist in patients whose primary diagnosis may be a personality disorder, a psychosis, or a psychophysiological autonomic and visceral condition. For more detailed information on the concept of anxiety we refer the reader to Chapters Eleven and Sixteen. In Chapter Seventeen the reader can find a discussion of ritualistic behavior and specific nursing intervention which make operational the concepts and principles underlying nursing care.

psychophysiologic autonomic and visceral disorders

The major concept which underlies the psychosomatic conditions is the idea that the mind and body function as a single entity in which there is a harmonious relationship and no dissociation of parts between the soma and the psyche. The concept emphasizes the interrelationship between the mind and the body. For example, have you ever had a toothache? How did you respond to people? Were you irritable? Short-tempered? Hypersensitive? Insensitive? If you were, you experienced an emotional response to physical pain. Have you ever had "butterflies in your stomach" before taking a test? Did you spend a restless night prior to the test or have to make frequent trips to the bathroom? The anxiety you experienced in relationship to the test produced the physiological response.

The second concept inherent in this classification is that feelings are discharged through the viscera and the specific physical illness which results serves as a channel for the expression of severe emotional stress. In these conditions, the feelings of inadequacy, insecurity, fear and anger are expressed through physiological processes rather than symbolically through behavior.

The more feeling the cerebral cortex is able to inhibit or repress, the more nervous energy must be directed downward through the autonomic nervous system and absorbed by the internal organs. This permits the repressed material to remain in the unconscious and thereby prevents it from becoming a conscious, emotionally painful experience. The resultant physical symptomotology differs from the symptoms seen in an anxiety reaction only because of their consistent, persistent impact on a particular organ producing structural changes that may be fatal if left untreated. Any organ may be affected, either because it may be biologically weak and therefore more susceptible or because a particular organ has a particular psychological significance or value for the individual. Regardless of which organ or body system is affected, the individual experiencing psychosomatic illness is responding to unconscious, emotional conflicts which, in turn, increase the amount of anxiety to a level where he can no longer meet his needs. The resultant phsyical illness is a direct expression of this conflict and permits a decrease in anxiety and gratification of needs through secondary gain.

The major principles and concepts pertinent to planning nursing intervention for patients with psychophysiologic autonomic and visceral disorders include the following.

Priority *must* be given to the alleviation of acute physical symptoms.

A calm, confident nursing approach is necessary to prevent reinforcement of secondary gain.

Feelings of security and personal worth are strengthened by a demonstration of respect.

Recognize that the nurse's feelings, behavior and understanding will influence the patient's response.

Individuals must be able to express their feelings (anger, fear, anxiety) in a calm, accepting atmosphere which does not negate their personal worth.

Relationships with others play a significant role in the development of ego identity.

To gain a more complete understanding of the psychosomatic process, the reader is directed to the following case study.

Mrs. Flora Jasper, a 69-year-old white female was readmitted to the hospital for treatment of her rheumatoid arthritis. Mrs. Jasper had a history of a refractory myocardial infarct, and an abdominal aortic aneurysm with repeated flareups of her arthritic condition. A student nurse was assigned to care for this patient for the purpose of establishing a therapeutic relationship. The student's primary goal was to assist the patient to deal more effectively with her arthritic condition. The student provided total in-hospital care and followed the patient after discharge for a three-month period. The student met with the patient and her husband for one hour each week in their home.

Flora and her husband Bill lived in a five-room apartment on the second floor of a deteriorating dwelling. They had been married for thirty-five years. It was the first marriage for Flora and the second for her husband. She reared two stepsons who no longer lived in the city. (When the oldest son left home he stole their life savings which they had had stuffed in their mattress.) The patient and her husband lived on a fixed income—a small retirement pension and Social Security. Their total monthly income was approximately $235.00. They had no hospital insurance plan and had accrued approximately $5,000 in hospital and related medical debts.

Flora had married her husband during the Depression. She was working in a dime store and most of her earnings went for support of other family members. Bill was divorced and had custody of his two little boys. She was a strict Catholic; he did not have any particular religious affiliation. At present Flora did not attend her church but her living room was filled with religious statues, pictures, icons, prayer beads, votive lights and crucifixes. She gave two reasons for not attending church—her physical condition prevented her and they did not have enough money to buy gas for their car.

When it was suggested that perhaps the parish priest could visit, she refused, saying she would be too ashamed to have him come to her house.

When the nurse visited each week Bill would meet the nurse on the corner and walk with her to the apartment. On entering the apartment, they always found Flora seated at one end of the kitchen table with a chair on either side in readiness to accommodate her husband and the nursing student. Flora dominated the conversation, relating many past events, sometimes repeating the situation over and over again. Occasionally she turned to her husband for confirmation and verification. The discussions revealed that their marital life had been and continued to be turbulent, argumentative and disruptive. She complained about Bill's inability to support them, the ingratitude of her two stepsons, regret about not having had a child of her own and repeatedly voiced bitter resentment over having been so foolish to marry Bill in the first place. During discourses Bill usually sat quietly with his head down. Once in awhile while Flora was particularly vitriolic he would contribute an angry retort or storm out of the room. As the tone of Flora's voice became more angry or when she spoke in a controlled, clipped, harsh manner there was a visible alteration in her joints. The inflammatory process would become acute with marked redness and swelling. If she got up to move from her chair, there were verbal expressions of pain.

On one particular occasion, the Jaspers were unable to focus on any of the issues previously discussed and the student realized that there was some problem that was apparently causing distress. After forty-five minutes of digression Bill finally said, "You want to know what it's all about! We had an argument last night about how the bedroom window should be opened. My bed is next to the window, it's hot and I like that breeze. Flora now, says the breeze bothers her and insists the window be open from the top, not the bottom!" He went on to describe how throughout the entire night they took turns opening and closing the window from the top and bottom. Flora said nothing, but the joints of her hands and knees turned bright red and visibly swelled. This observable change was brought to Flora's attention. The nurse attempted to help the patient see the connection between the felt anger and her physical condition. With the resolution of the problem, there was a corresponding resolution of the inflammatory process.

A gradual reduction from the pressures of daily living along with a progressively more effective verbalization of angry feelings and the development of alternative coping devices including some rudimentary ability to compromise resulted in an appreciable decrease in the number and severity of inflammatory flareups.

The psychosomatic illnesses are often the most covertly insidious of the psychopathologies. Because of the obvious medical problems resulting from sustained, prolonged emotional stresses and conflicts, it is easy to overlook the psychological etiology of the illness. The preceding case history demonstrates the necessity for critical, accurate observation and recognition of those overt, sometimes masked, behavioral displays, both verbal and non-verbal, which assist in differential diagnosis. In addition to those concepts and principles previously outlined, the nurse must always be alert to those behaviors which lend themselves to the identification of the total diagnostic clinical picture.

personality disorders

The personality disorders can best be described as a disorganized way of living. They are probably the most challenging and the least understood of the psychiatric disorders. Unlike many of the other diagnostic categories the personality disorders originate from a cathexis of lifelong experiences resulting in basic disturbances in the individual's ability to interact appropriately with society within the context of societal norms. Since the personality disorders demonstrate a repetitive pattern of behavior which manifests specific deficits within the personality structure, the individual experiences problems in living rather than specific symptoms as was seen with the psychoneurotic or psychosomatic disorders.

The type of maladjusted behavior which is evidenced indicates that the observable pathology is outwardly directed toward and against others. Significantly, the results of the pathological process does not seem to affect the individual with feelings of anxiety, guilt or depression. Because of its lifelong, deeply ingrained, and persistent nature, causation is attributed to faulty or arrested emotional development during the first three years of life where there has been apparent interference with the development of adequate social control or superego formation. Therefore, during early childhood experiences the individual has most likely been deprived of satisfactory gratification of the basic needs of love, security, trust and responsibility.

The characteristic symptom pattern associated with personality disorders incorporates one or more of the following.

Poor or marginal interpersonal relationships.

Severe limited ability to feel or experience emotions (patient is often described as "cold" or "unfeeling").

Easily distractable.

Poor self-motivation.

Marked lack of persistence except in areas of self-gratification.

Limited stress tolerance.

Impulsivity.

Verbally and/or physically explosive especially when crossed.

Poor discriminative and reflective judgment.

Fails to profit from experience.

Lacks foresight.

Distorted or absent moral code or value system.

Behavior is generally manipulative, self-defeating and destructive.

With each succeeding revision of the nomenclature there has been marked reorganization and realignment of the specific diagnostic categories included in this section. This diagnostic category includes a myriad of conditions covering a wide array of personality, character and behavioral maladjustments in living. We refer the reader to the reference and suggested reading material at the end of the chapter for more detailed information on the specific conditions that were identified in Table 14-1.

The case history of Paul Miller is a typical example of two of the clinical conditions seen in this broad diagnostic category. His diagnoses are episodic excessive drinking and antisocial personality.

Paul Miller is a 19-year-old black male who was admitted to a state hospital after having severely beaten both of his parents while under the influence of alcohol. His parents reported that, "He was always a problem" and was continuously in and out of trouble at school. At the age of 14, Paul was with his friend in a stolen car when they were stopped by the police who, according to the patient, later "beat them" and brought them to a juvenile detention home. Subsequently, Paul was placed on probation for two and a half years. Since that time Paul developed an animosity toward the police and believes that the police are "doing wrong and not doing justice to the people." The patient has had several confrontations with the police but he refused to elaborate on the specific incidents. However, in talking with the nurses on the ward, he did relate portions of some of these experiences. He admits to having robbed the homes of some elderly people across town. He stated that in his conscience he does not feel that there is anything wrong with this, "After all, I didn't steal from our neighbors." He further commented that, "This is a dog-eat-dog world. I was brought up on the streets." He admitted that he started to drink at the age of 16. Since that time he has had many episodes of excessive drinking and that when he came home he was, according to his parents, violent, hostile and unmanageable. One year ago, he related that he struck his father for the first time and later he also struck his mother. His mother stated that she is "scared of him." A few months ago, Paul left his parent's home and went to live in an apartment with a friend. He worked sporadically at various kinds of odd jobs but never for very long. Paul describes himself as "a good worker, who deserves more than what I get paid" and "a good friend with people I get along with."

His parents voiced concern about their son's behavior, stating that they had tried different ways to reach him in an effort to prevent his drinking habit but that they were not successful. They thought they had the solution when he came home last week, drunk and threatening. They called the police. But by the time the police had arrived, Paul had severely beaten both his parents. Paul was taken to the city jail and later transferred to the hospital. His parents were treated at a nearby hospital emergency room and released. They have hopes that perhaps this hospitalization will help him to find a morally and socially acceptable way of life.

In the hospital, the patient made new friends and became more interested in politics. He made several statements about the conditions in the United States and his room is full of political literature, most of it Leftist, for example, Quotations from Chairman Mao Tse-tung, Report to the Ninth

National Congress of the Communist Party of China, and Mass Line Newspaper of the American Communist Workers Movement. He stated that he is trying to find a life on his own, that he is not yet a Communist but is learning and trying to understand what is going on.

He wrote a letter to his parents in which he tried to convince them of his new political views and tried to explain what these things mean to him. He wrote, "The nation is run by the government and the government is run by the rich. All of the masses of the working people are the backbone of the country. In a matter of years, not many, there will be a revolution and there will be a great change in government and all Fascist courts, police, judges, and other unrealistic forces trained in using the great masses of the people then will no longer be."

In the same letter, he describes some of his experiences at the hospital: "When I inquired the purpose of the pills which they had given to me, they would say they were 'to keep me calm and from being nervous and upset'. Since, they have said, 'Don't you sleep much better since you have taken the pills in the daytime?'—although I have taken none all of this time, but two."

During various therapy sessions Paul's mood changed from time to time. Sometimes he was very cooperative and friendly, talking freely, logically and coherently about his personal problems and his personal life history. When his drinking habits were discussed, he repeatedly stated he felt he was old enough and adult enough to take the responsibility of this and said he is able to stop himself from becoming drunk but also says he "has pleasure from being drunk and I want to do it again." He describes himself as "a lumpen proletarian who belongs to the proletariat but prefers an easy way of life if possible with luxury, pleasure, etc." He says he "likes to have everything the best." If he has to choose, he wants to have "the best car, the best home, the best suit, the best shoes, and everything the best. I want to enjoy a family, and have at least one boy and a daughter, but no more than four children." He says that he does not like a formal way of education and does not like to work in a factory—he prefers to be "the man who delivers and carries things on the truck." He further characterizes himself as having "a hot temper and one who acts easily and quickly." He demonstrated this aspect of his personality in several of the sessions by jumping up, waving his arms and talking in a loud voice when the topics focused on issues or subjects he disliked.

He enjoys going to occupational and recreational therapy and spends much of his time talking politics with other patients, especially those younger than himself. Periodically, he insists that he has to be released as soon as possible. He is becoming slightly more critical of his drinking habits and states he is sorry for hitting his parents. He believes he is ready to go home, return to his family and try to start a new life.

On initial encounter, those individuals who manifest personality disorders give the impression of being intelligent, charming, pleasant, friendly and nonchalant people. However, closer scrutiny of the behavior and verbal comments such as those made by Paul Miller in the above case presentation indicate that the facade is often misleading.

In planning intervention for patients with personality disorders the nurse will find the following concepts and principles helpful:

The nurse-patient relationship must incorporate learning experiences directed toward maturation.

Intervention must be guided by the consistent use of rational authority which permits freedom and experimentation within specified limits.

Limit setting is the application of a consistent set of expectations which guide the patient toward the development of self-control.

The nursing responsibility requires provision for experimentation coupled with assistance toward realistic self-evaluation by the patient.

The nurse must recognize that the patient will frequently attempt to place responsibility for the satisfaction of his needs on others.

Inability to recognize and/or to control personal feelings toward the patient will impede the therapeutic process.

In summary, the nurse should keep in mind that those individuals afflicted with personality disorders seldom see themselves as needing help. They view themselves as being in step and consider the rest of the world in contention with them. They tend to be consummate actors attempting to fool others and in the process, end up fooling themselves instead. They play at life and living, many times never fully realizing what it is that they are missing. Their plight is sad for they miss one of life's most unique experiences—loving and being loved.

psychoses

Psychoses are a flight from reality into an inner world of fantasy—a world which is at once bizarre, frightening, overwhelming and yet, apparently infinitely more bearable than the "real world." The psychotic experiences such inner pain and conflict that his patterns of thinking, feeling and acting become grossly distorted. Frequently, these exaggerated and disturbed manifestations are not only frightening to the individual but they also frighten those with whom he comes in contact. The psychotic individual may be described as a person who is out of tune with the rest of society—someone who just doesn't make sense to others. The psychotic individual is one who overreacts, underreacts or reacts uniquely and unexpectedly to the general demands of living.

Psychoses are major mental disorders whose chief characteristic is gross deterioration in ego functioning. Severe personality disintegration and disorganization is manifested through disorientation in the cognitive and sensory spheres, withdrawal and isolation from the environment and offensive or bizarre behavior that is often accompanied by pronounced regression. There are several diagnostic categories within the classification of psychotic disorders (see Table 14-1).

schizophrenia

Schizophrenia is probably the most prevalant of the psychotic disorders due to its early onset and chronic nature. Schizophrenia represents a group of reactions whose chief characteristics appear to be an inability to formulate reality relationships, disturbances in the boundaries of self-image along with distortions in the affective and cognitive domains. The four primary symptoms connected with the schizophrenic disorders are ambivalence, autism, looseness of associations and affective disturbances. The predominant behavior pattern exhibited is withdrawal.

The schizophrenic patient is unable to cope with the problems of living. His use of ego defenses is often ineffective and inappropriate which results in intense and overwhelming anxiety. As the anxiety mounts the patient isolates himself from others and displays a lack of concern for social demands in an attempt to ward off possible anticipated rejection from others, thus evidencing a widening social distance which progresses to the pathological state of loneliness. Characteristically, the schizophrenic's fantasy world is dominated by delusions of persecution, auditory hallucinations and preoccupation with body functionings.

Many theories have been postulated regarding the possible cause or causes of schizophrenia; however, a review of the current literature reveals that despite the number of studies that have been conducted, no single cause has as yet been identified. The most likely theory is that of multiple causation, taking into account such factors as the individual's vulnerability and sensitivity to stress; the type of personality the individual is or was prior to onset; the specific modes of adaptation the individual uses in the stress situation; the type of social, cultural and economic background which influenced his development; his biophysiological and chemical makeup and familial hereditary factors.

The complexity of the symptom picture of schizophrenia has resulted in the identification of numerous subtypes. Included among these subtypes are the following.

simple

This type of schizophrenia is characterized by early onset, usually in adolescence, in which there is a gradual reduction in interest, an increase in apathy and a lessening of social relationships. Communication is on a concrete and superficial level. Simple schizophrenics appear to be aloof or peculiar and are frequently described by others as being eccentric and chronically irritable. Hallucinations and delusions are generally not a part of the symptom picture. This type of individual lives a marginal and transient type of existence and if employed, can carry out simple routine tasks under direct supervision. Often, the simple schizophrenic resists efforts to change or alter his routine existence. His behavior, although withdrawn and slightly bizarre seldom necessitates hospitalization.

hebephrenic

This type of schizophrenic disorder demonstrates a more severe disintegration of the personality. The background of the patient often reveals a history of numerous peculiar mannerisms, overscrupulousness about trivial matters, and preoccupation with religious or philosophical issues. The hebephrenic patient experiences disorganized thinking, a shallow and markedly inappropriate affect accompanied by excessive giggling, silliness and severe regressive behavior. Hallucinations and delusions are common and are transient, unsystematized and bizarre. Usually the hebephrenic patient will display obscene behavior and demonstrate a frank absence of any modesty or sense of shame. In addition, this individual is subjected to impulsive, explosive outbursts of angry, hostile feelings and displays temper tantrums which are generally in response to the individual's fantasy life.

catatonic

This clinical condition appears suddenly and is commonly observed to be of two subtypes—catatonic excitement and catatonic stupor. Typically, there may be alterations or swings between these two subtypes. Catatonic excitement is characterized by hyperactivity, that is, excessive and sometimes violent motor activity. Typical behavior includes marked agitation, impulsive and explosive acting out. Catatonic stupor is characterized by a loss of animation, mutism, negativism and waxy flexibility. The patient is unable to function independently. He will remain motionless for long periods of time and seldom responds to verbal commands. However, while in this apparently detached state the individual does not lose awareness of his environment even though he demonstrates no obvious external response.

paranoid

The paranoid type generally becomes apparent in adult life. Characteristically, the patient's life pattern has been dominated by hostility, suspicion and distrust. The patient's autistic manifestations are predominantly those of persecutory or grandiose delusions and auditory hallucinations of an accusatory and/or threatening nature. Much of the patient's ideation centers around sexual and religious content. In this type, regression is less pronounced with a corresponding ability to sustain some semblance of personality organization and attention to the maintenance of physical appearance.

schizo-affective

This subtype reflects a mixture of the disorganized thought process of schizophrenia with the exaggerated and extreme feeling states of elation or depression characteristic of the manic-depressive. Diagnosis is made on the presence of these profound feelings which are significantly different from the schizophrenic's usual or general symptoms of indifference or apathy.

childhood schizophrenia

This clinical condition is usually observed prior to the onset of puberty. Apparently onset is closely connected with a traumatic incident within the family living experience such as the birth of a sibling or abrupt disruption in the mother-child relationship. Withdrawal and regression occur, primitive speech and communication patterns predominate and behavior is primarily autistic with a retreat into fantasy accompanied by bizarre gestures and mannerisms. Since normal growth and development includes a rich fantasy life, it is often difficult to identify hallucinatory and delusional systems. In childhood schizophrenia one notices very pronounced object relationships as opposed to the normal and usual developing interpersonal relationships.

For further details to supplement this brief overview of the schizophrenic process, dynamics and subclassification the reader is referred to the suggested readings at the end of the chapter.

In addition, Chapter 20 is a complete account of a patient with a diagnosis of schizophrenia, paranoid type. This chapter describes the family constellation, identifies developing symptomatology and precipitating stress factors which led to psychiatric hospitalization. Chapter Twenty-one is a further elaboration and contains the completed nursing assessment and subsequent intervention.

manic-depressive psychosis

Manic-depressive psychosis is a psychotic reaction characterized by severe recurring mood swings which may range from profound depression to unbridled elation wtih corresponding behavioral manifestations of underactivity or overactivity. Subclassifications are based on the predominant mood and are commonly referred to as manic type, depressed type or circular type.

This condition usually manifests itself between the ages of twenty to thirty-five. Current theory supports the idea that genetic factors may be involved along with some biochemical or physiologic alterations. Analytic theory places emphasis on unmet oral needs, self-hatred and loss of self-esteem. It is commonly accepted that the feelings of aggression and hostility of the manic-depressive are in response to threats to his security and self-esteem. The outward expression of aggression results in manic behavior while the inward direction of aggression results in depressive behavior.

Unlike the schizophrenic, the manic-depressive individual maintains a better integrated self-system and his total functioning is less bizarre and distorted. To further compare and contrast the significant differences between schizophrenia and manic-depressive psychoses, the following outline in Table 14-3 will assist the reader in distinguishing the etiologic, symptomologic and dynamic differences in these two prevalent and frequently encountered disorders.

The following two case presentations serve to provide the reader with a picture of the manic and depressed types of the manic-depressive psychosis.

situation I

Present Illness: Kathryn Howard is a 24-year-old, white, married woman who was admitted to a state hospital for the second time on a voluntary basis. She was first admitted to the state hospital in early February but was subsequently transferred to a small private hospital. After one week in that facility she was taken home by her husband and remained there until her present admission in early March. At this time, she was agitated,

TABLE 14-3
GENERAL COMPARISON OF THE SCHIZOPHRENIC AND MANIC-DEPRESSIVE PSYCHOSES

Elements for Comparison	Schizophrenia	Manic-Depressive Psychosis	
		Manic Phase	Depressive Phase
1) Prepsychotic Personality	Introvertive. Aloof. Daydreams. Shy and indifferent. Rejecting. Emotionally detached.	Extrovertive. Overtly aggressive. Manipulative. Confident and friendly. Sensitive. Pronounced feeling of well-being.	Unobtrusive. Passively aggressive. Rigid and fearful. Timid and retiring. Sensitive. Pronounced feeling of sadness.
2) Causes	Multiple causes. Most likely related to psychological, sociocultural, organic and hereditary factors.	Traumatic Stress. Long standing unresolved conflict. Poorly developed and integrated ego boundaries. Unresolved diffuse anger and hostility. Repeated failure in early life to measure up to parental expectations.	Loss of significant others or objects.
3) Dynamics	Withdrawal from reality. Preoccupation with fantasy. Fear of rejection. Regression to complete dependency.	Unmet needs during infancy given rise to feelings of insecurity and dependency with resultant ambivalence. Confidence and self-assurance is defense against dependency. Represses hostility and guilt in effort to seek approval from others.	Real or imaginary loss perceived as rejection. Repressed hostility and hatred turned inward as a result of rigid superego. Penance in the form of guilt feelings for aggressive and hostile feelings. Denial of aggression produces

TABLE 14-3 (continued)

Elements for Comparison	Schizophrenia	Manic-Depressive Psychosis	
		Manic Phase	Depressive Phase
3) Dynamics (continued)		Unrealistic expectations of self give rise to feelings of inferiority and inadequacy. Flight into reality. Attacks external environment. Uses rationalization and projection.	helplessness and hopelessness.
4) Symptoms a) Cognitive process	Associative looseness. Autistic or magical thinking. Concrete rather than abstract. Vague and neologistic. Illogical. Blocking. Depersonalization. Hallucinations. Perseverance. Incoherence. Religiosity.	Flight of ideas. Circumstantiality. Grandiose delusions. Distractability. Rhyming. Punning. Clang association. Absence of self-criticism. Poor judgment.	Poverty of ideas. Retardation of thought process. Self-accusatory and somatic delusions. Confusion and perplexity. Impairment of concentration and memory. Excessive preoccupation with a particularly personal meaningful life event. Suicidal preoccupation.
b) Multisensory integration	Inappropriate affect. Blunted or flattened affect. Inadequate, inconsistent or exaggerated affect.	Euphoric, effusive, elated. Volatile and erratic. Aggressive, irritable and self-exaltive.	Despondency, despair. Gloom, pessimism. Unworthiness, guilt. Inadequacy, inferiority.

TABLE 14-3 (continued)

Elements for Comparison	Schizophrenia	Manic-Depressive Psychosis	
		Manic Phase	Depressive Phase
4) Symptoms b) Multisensory integration (continued)	Ambivalence. Indifference. Distrust. Shallowness. Anxiety. Loneliness. Apathy.	Increasing intensity of pseudo-positive feeling states. Omnipotence and omniscience.	Helplessness and hopeless-ness. Bitterness and anger. Fear, loneliness. Anxiety.
c) Psychomotor activity	Withdrawn. Negativistic. Ritualistic. Automatism. Impulsive. Regressive. Posturing.	Hyperactive. Boisterous, teasing, meddle-some. Arrogant and pompous. Sarcastic, insulting and caustic. Irritable, abusive or violent. Exhibitionalistic, vulgar and pro-fane. Overtly seductive and obscene. Wakeful.	Underactive or agitated. Marked fatigue. Lack of appetite. Weight loss. Early morning wakefulness. Suicidal gestures. Lassitude. Bored. Crying.
5) Concepts and Principles for Nursing Care.	Maintain focus of patient on re-ality. The primary goal of the inter-personal relationship is to build trust.	Exaggerated responses to stimuli necessitates a physical and emotional environment that is nonstimulating.	Provide for safety and protec-tion against self-destructive be-havior. Survival for the patient depends

TABLE 14-3 (continued)

Elements for Comparison	Schizophrenia	Manic-Depressive Psychosis	
		Manic Phase	Depressive Phase
5) Concepts and Principles for Nursing Care (continued)	Rejection and resistance are maneuvers which should be met by nurse with acceptance, consistency and persistence.	Maintain neutrality and objectivity in light of patient hyperactive behavior.	On the meeting of his basic needs.
	Due to the patient's limited capacity for intimacy, the nurse must proceed slowly in planning for socialization.	A firm, honest, consistent approach is an effective means of dealing with manipulative behavior.	Monitor environment for potential hazards.
	Frustration tolerance is minimal, therefore simple activities with limited concentration and no competition are most effective.	Limit interpersonal contacts. Hyperactivity leads to exhaustion.	Keep patient under close observation. Nursing care should focus on lessening the patient's feelings of guilt and increasing self-esteem.
	Activities and personal contacts should be directed to increasing self-esteem and feelings of adequacy.	Set limits to prevent injury to self and others. Instructions should be clear and concise.	Planned scheduled activities are needed to increase social contacts, distract preoccupation with self and lessen the feelings of hopelessness and helplessness.
	Security operations should be supported until such time that the patient learns new ways of adapting.	Recognize feelings and responses to the patient which tend to maintain pathological behavior.	A subtle, pleasant, interested approach will reinforce a sense of dignity and worth. Allow the patient to respond in his own time.
	The nurse must exercise judgment in determining how much the patient is able to do for self and how much the nurse needs to do for him.	Allow for verbal expressions of hostility without punitive or judgmental reactions. Maintain interpersonal and environmental distance which allows the patient freedom of movement. Remain calm, poised, unhurried and patient.	Support the patient with verbal encouragement. Worthwhile menial tasks enable the individual to rid himself of guilt and allow him to feel a sense of accomplishment.

overtalkative, delusional and the presence of hallucinations was suspected.

Past History: Kathryn was born in Chicago and has lived in Illinois all of her life except for the last six months which was spent in Lancaster, Pennsylvania. She is the oldest of four. Kathryn finished high school and during her admission interview stated that she did not like school and had never made good grades except in English. Kathryn married at eighteen and held a variety of jobs until her son was born about three years ago. Her husband, who is twenty-seven, is somewhat effeminate and immature. They dated each other since Kathryn was in the ninth grade and neither had had any previous dating experience. Kathryn is Protestant and her husband, Joe, is Jewish, and for this reason both sets of parents have always disapproved of the marriage. Joe had been working as a disc jockey in Lancaster but lost his job because of his wife's behavior and at present is unemployed, receiving welfare. Now they live alternately with each set of parents. Kathryn's mother is forty-one; her father, fifty-one, is a diabetic, has had recurrent skin cancer and has just recently had surgery. One brother, age twenty-three, has asthma, is retarded, lives at home and works in a laundry close by. Two other siblings, a sister, 13, and a brother, 4, are in good health and live with their parents.

Appearance and Behavior: Kathryn is a well-developed, adequately nourished woman who looks and acts like a 15-year-old. She is oriented in all three spheres. Her speech is rapid, constant, irrelevant and she speaks with a "little girl voice." She demonstrates a flight of ideas, delusions and a labile mood which alternates between euphoria and slight depression. She talks of getting pregnant from men who slipped into her hospital bed and raped her. She says, "My husband is a fag. My mother didn't give me the right attention and it has to come out some way. I think I might be a man. I have a large Adam's apple. I am writing a book. People send me messages. I can predict for the President of the United States. The President is a communist. I have supernatural powers. I am helping all these girls. God talks to me. I know nobody believes me."

Kathryn's memory is intact, she displays no insight and her judgment is impaired. She is hyperactive, spends a great deal of time pacing, shouting orders, advising others and sleeps about four hours per night.

situation II

Present Illness: George Garner is a 44-year-old, black, married male who was admitted to a state hospital for the first time. On admission he was in a state of psychomotor retardation, depressed and responded only to direct questions in a whispering monotone.

Past History: George was born in Birmingham, Alabama. His family moved to the Cleveland area when he was three years old. He is the third of nine siblings. His two older brothers and a younger sister were killed in an automobile accident fifteen years ago. The remaining three brothers and two sisters are married and well. His parents are both dead.

George graduated from college, earned a teaching certificate and is currently a high school principal. He met his wife, Mildred, while in college and they were married shortly after their graduation. They have no children.

He was promoted to his present position just two months ago. For a month prior to admission, he had shown an increasing inability to perform his duties. His lack of initiative and depressed emotional state was noticed by his wife, family, students and colleagues.

His history revealed one other psychiatric hospitalization when he was 30 years old, just one month after his automobile accident. His wife reports that he has had periodic "fits of depression" where he would cry, wring his hands, and refuse to eat but, "they didn't last long." She says that his usual behavior is quiet, retiring and he is never very happy. His wife further related that after the death of each of his parents he became very morose and frequently expressed the thought that he should die. Mildred stated that she thought this episode was like all the rest and that it would go away after awhile, but she really became concerned when she found him standing motionless in the middle of the bathroom holding a straight razor in his hand. He would not respond to her or tell her what he was doing. It was at this point that she called his brother and together they brought him to the hospital.

Appearance and Behavior: George is a tall, thin almost emaciated man who looks and acts like an "old man." In the hospital, he refuses to eat, sleeps an average of four hours a night, and replies in barely audible monosyllables when questioned. He usually stands or sits with head bowed, eyes downcast, has a dejected facial expression and will not join in activities wtih other patients or personnel. He is oriented to reality. However, he expresses a self-accusatory delusional system in which he blames himself for the deaths of his brothers and sister in an auto accident in which he was the driver.

The above case histories, although markedly different in terms of social history and presenting symptoms, have a common denominator which is displayed through affective and behavioral patterns that represent an exaggerated aggressive response to living. In Situation I, Kathryn's response is externalized onto the environment resulting in loud, hyperactive and overtly aggressive dominating behavior. In Situation II, George's aggression is turned inward on himself resulting in rejection of the worth-while self, overwhelming guilt and self-punishment.

acute and chronic brain syndromes

Acute and chronic brain syndromes comprise a vast group of psychiatric disorders which are primarily caused by some agent or process that results in impaired cerebral functioning. The major factor which distinguishes an acute syndrome from a chronic syndrome is the potential for reversibility of the pathophysiological damage to the brain. When cerebral impairment is reversible the syndrome is classified as "acute"; when the condition is irreversible, the syndrome is identified as "chronic."

Acute brain syndromes may result from infections, traumatic injuries, metabolic imbalance, severe cardiac disease or from the toxicity associated with alcohol, drugs or poisons. The acute condition is usually sudden in onset and of a brief duration. Generally, the prognosis for an individual diagnosed as having acute brain syndrome is good if the underlying etiological factors can be isolated and treated. Treatment most often results in remission. However, if the severity and degree of damage is extensive, chronicity or death follows.

Chronic brain syndromes may arise from the same etiological factors as do the acute. However, the most common chronic brain syndromes result from the pathophysiological change and deterioration produced by the normal aging process. In these conditions onset is usually slow and insidious. In addition, there may well be a more pronounced and diffuse disintegration in the individual's personality.

A common organic syndrome is characteristic of this very broad diagnostic category. The primary symptoms associated with the basic organic syndrome consist of impairment of both recent and remote memory with remote memory remaining fairly well intact for a longer period of time; marked deficiency in immediate recall and disorientation in the three spheres—time, place and person; and gross impairment of intellectual functioning involving decreased comprehension, inability to solve problems or learn new facts, behaviors or activities. All of these are found in any one of the diagnostic conditions, although the degree of severity is not necessarily the same for each.

Concommitantly, secondary symptoms which involve lability of affect, disorganized thought content and aberrant behavior may be superimposed on the existing syndrome. The broad secondary symptom spectrum may include any combination of apathy, depression or euphoria; marked anxiety and agitation; confabulation, fabrication or paranoid ideation; withdrawal and regression; and hyperactivity or psychomotor retardation. The secondary symptoms observed in each individual case are considered to represent the individual's exaggerated response or reaction of his basic personality to his mental and physical disability. Therefore, the specific symptomatology apparently is related to the individual's premorbid personality, pre-existing patterns or modes of adjustment, socioeconomic, cultural and environmental situation as well as the extent of his individual and group interpersonal relationships. A well-integrated individual can withstand organic brain damage better than a person who has manifested a rigid, immature, or other mental, emotional or psychological disability or inadequacy. Thus, the great variability of individual response to illness accounts for the diversity of secondary symptomotology.

The following two case studies detail the development and progression of the most commonly encountered acute and chronic brain syndromes—delirium tremens and cerebral arteriosclerosis:

situation III

Mr. Edward Nolen, age 47, was admitted to a general hospital with a diagnosis of acute appendicitis. Within forty-eight hours following surgery, Mr. Nolen displayed increasing restlessness and agitation. He was found trying to wash his face and hands with the water from his ice pitcher, and when he saw the nurse he wanted to know if she could do something about the "room service in this hotel." He asked the nurse to order a "shot and a beer" for him and as soon as he finished getting dressed he would be glad to take her to dinner in the hotel dining room, that is, if she could assure him that the service in the dining room was better than the room service. When the nurse proceeded to explain that he was in the hospital, he became angry and verbally abusive. He picked up the phone and tried to place a call to the "head man in charge" to get this "interfering female" out of his room. Shortly afterwards, Mr. Nolen shouted for someone to come and get "these terrible creatures off his bed." In his agitation and in his attempt to get away, he pulled off his dressing, disconnected his i.v., and ruptured his incision.

Emergency intervention included the immediate return to surgery for incisioned repair and the planning for close, continuous observation and care of his post surgery. His caloric intake was increased, Librium was ordered to alleviate and prevent further agitation, and a Vitamin B complex regime was instituted. Within three days after the second surgery Mr. Nolen was no longer disoriented, nor was there any evidence of hallucinations or delusions. When his sensorium cleared, the patient was distressed and apologetic about his behavior. Both he and his wife stated that although he was once a heavy drinker, he had joined Alcoholics Anonymous five years ago and has not had a drink since. They had been convinced that this episode could not happen again.

situation IV

Mrs. Dorothy Snelling is a 74-year-old white female who was admitted to the Greenbriar Nursing Home at the request of her daughter Nancy. In talking with the staff nurse, Nancy described her mother as a woman who had been very independent and who had taken great pride in her personal appearance. Over the past four years Nancy noticed obvious changes. For example, Mrs. Snelling had trouble remembering where she put things such as her eyeglasses, pocketbook and dentures and had on one occasion put the coffee pot in the refrigerator. She had been in the habit of walking the dog every afternoon and lately was having difficulty finding her way back home, so that Nancy would have to drive around the neighborhood looking for her. Gradually her behavior became more erratic and unpredictable. Six months ago Mrs. Snelling gave a valuable piece of jewelry to the boy next door because she believed he was her son John. John was killed in the Second World War. Over the next few months she became more irritable and demanding and would often accuse Nancy of trying to get rid of her. She lost interest in her appearance, was reluctant and even resistive to bathe and flatly refused to let Nancy wash and set her hair. Lately, the neighbors reported to Nancy that Mrs. Snelling spent much of her time standing inside the front door, yelling at them whenever they appeared outside. Last week Mrs. Snelling found her way to the corner drugstore where she purchased a package of Rit Dye and colored her own very white hair a bright red. Two days ago when Nancy came home she found the house filled with smoke. Mrs. Snelling was ironing and had placed the hot iron on the dining room chair when she finished and had forgotten to turn it off. Nancy found her sitting calmly in the kitchen reading the newspaper, completely oblivious of the hole in the chair or the smoke-filled dining room. This event finally convinced Nancy that her mother could no longer safely manage on her own.

The preliminary admitting diagnosis of cerebral arteriosclerosis was made.

Most often initial treatment for an individual with an organic brain syndrome takes place in a general hospital setting since the presenting symptoms or basic etiological factors produce marked physiological change. In this setting, the initial focus of care is twofold. Whether one is dealing with a patient with delirium tremens, meningitis, arteriosclerotic heart disease, multiple sclerosis, or Parkinson's syndrome, the care is directed toward alleviating the phsyical symptomology where the primary aim is maintenance of life support systems and return to physiological equilibrium. Concurrently, equal emphasis is given to sustaining the psychological coping mechanisms already in operation. Such emotional and psychological emphasis contributes to the preservation of the individual's psychological need system, safeguards personal integrity, provides emotional security and curtails further personality disintegration.

Concepts and principles upon which nursing intervention is based include:

Basic needs for survival take precedence.

Any threat to self-esteem and self-respect can retard progress toward health.

Feelings of self-esteem increase in direct proportion to the amount of respect the individual receives.

Feelings of inadequacy, uselessness and helplessness can be mitigated.

Progressive destruction of cerebral tissue produces an inability to adapt responsively to changing conditions or stress, leading to confusion and irritability.

Sensory and social deprivation increases regressive behavior.

Work and social activities serve to maintain self-esteem and enhance reality orientation.

Gratification of the interpersonal needs for affection, recognition and control promotes movement toward the maintenance of emotional equilibrium.

Provision for personal satisfaction, comfort and dignity are the basis for fostering self-worth.

Minimizing an individual's exposure to new people or new experiences will decrease the potential for adverse reactions.

Consistency in the attitudes and behavior of health care personnel promotes security and provides reassurance.

Careful, well-planned and structured routines will minimize progression of the disability and maximize opportunities for rehabilitation.

This chapter is a concise synthesis of predominant psychopathology. It provides essential, relevant, factual information. It serves as a basis for distinguishing and differentiating between pathological phenomenon. It is a fundamental frame of reference designed to promote the nurse's understanding of psychopathology operational within individual patients. From this base the nurse should be able to participate intelligently with other members of the interdisciplinary team.

As an essential care provider the nurse is apt to find that patients do not always conform to the textbook picture. People are unique and defy classification, categorization and labeling. In fact, patients usually manifest a crisscrossing of symptomotology. Thus, the textbook serves only as a frame of reference since it is with the individual patient, his concerns, needs and problems with which the nurse must deal. Knowledge of the pathological process is important only insofar as it contributes to furthering the nurse's assessment or appraisal of the individual patient's need system.

The focus of nursing is *always* on the patient and not on his illness. It is not the diagnostic label that receives treatment, intervention and recognition, but rather, the individual who is suffering, cries out in his loneliness, lives with overwhelming anxiety, cannot differentiate the real from the unreal, or experiences self-defeating helplessness and hopelessness. The nurse's primary task is to assist those in distress to establish pathways which lead to healthier, happier and more successful adjustments in living.

suggested readings

Aaronson, Lauren S. "Alienation and Paranoia." *Perspectives in Psychiatric Care,* Vol. 15 No. 1 (1977).

Alfano, Genrose, J. "There Are No Routine Patients." *American Journal of Nursing,* Vol. 75 No. 10 (October, 1975), 1804-1807.

Almeida, Elza M., and Chapman, A. H. *The Interpersonal Basis of Psychiatric Nursing.* G. P. Putnam's Sons: New York, 1972.

Anderson, Nancy P. "Suicide in Schizophrenia." *Perspectives in Psychiatric Care,* Vol. 11 No. 3 (1973), 106-112.

Arnold, Helen M. "Four A's: A Guide to One-to-one Relationships." *American Journal of Nursing,* Vol. 76 No. 6 (June, 1976), 941-943.

Bahara, Robert J. "The Potential For Suicide." *American Journal of Nursing,* Vol. 75 No. 10 (October, 1975), 1782-1788.

Burnside, Irene Mortenson. "Listen To The Aged." *American Journal of Nursing,* Vol. 75 No. 10 (October, 1975), 1800-1803.

Caplan, Gerald, *Principles of Preventive Psychiatry.* Basic Books, Inc.: New York, 1964.

Carlson, Carolyn E., and Blackwell, Betty, eds. *Behavioral Concepts and Nursing Intervention.* 2d ed. J. B. Lippincott Company: Philadelphia, 1978.

Clancy, John; Noyes, Russell Jr.; and Travis, Terry A. "The Hostile-Dependent Personality." *Nursing Digest,* Vol. 3 No. 2 (March/April, 1975), 21-22.

Cospers, Bonnie. "The Yo-Yo Factor in Chronic Illness." *Nursing Forum,* Vol. 13 No. 2 (1974), 207-211.

Eaton, Merrill T., Jr.; Peterson, Margaret H.; and Davis, James A. *Psychiatry.* 3d ed. Medical Examination Publishing Company, Inc.: Flushing, New York, 1976.

Field, William E., and Wilkerson, Sandra. "Religiosity as a Psychiatric Symptom." *Perspectives in Psychiatric Care,* Vol. 11 No. 3 (1973), 99-105.

Finkelman, Anita Ward. "The Nurse Therapist: Outpatient Crisis Intervention With the Chronic Psychiatric Patient." *Journal of Psychiatric Nursing and Mental Health Services,* Vol. 15 No. 8 (August, 1977), 27-32.

Fitzgerald, Ray G., and Long, Imelda. "Seclusion in the Treatment and Management of Severely Disturbed Manic and Depressed Patients." *Perspectives in Psychiatric Care,* Vol. II No. 2 (1973), 59-63.

Freedman, Alfred, ed. *Comprehensive Textbook of Psychiatry.* Williams and Wilkins Company: Baltimore, 1975.

Horowitz, June Andrews. "Sexual Difficulties as Indicators of Broader Personal and Interpersonal Problems." *Perspectives of Psychiatric Care,* Vol. 16 No. 2 (March/April 1978), 66-69.

Irving, Susan. *Basic Psychiatric Nursing.* W. B. Saunders Co.: Philadelphia, 1973.

Johnson, C. Warner; Snibbe, John R.; and Evans, Leonard A., eds. *Basic Psychopathology: A Programmed Text.* Spectrum Publications, Inc.: New York, 1975.

Kahn, Alice. "Stranger in the World of I.C.U." *American Journal of Nursing,* Vol. 75 No. 11 (November, 1975), 2072-2025.

Knapp, Terry J., and Peterson, Linda Whitney. "Behavior Analysis for Nursing and Somatic Disorders." *Nursing Research,* Vol. 26 No. 4 (July/August 1977), 281-287.

Kolb, Lawrence C. *Noyes' Modern Clinical Psychiatry.* 7th ed. W. B. Saunders Company: Philadelphia, 1968.

Lynch, Vincent J., and Lynch, Mary Theresa. "The Borderline Personality." *Perspectives in Psychiatric Care,* Vol. 15 No. 2 (February, 1977), 72-77.

Manfreda, Marguerite Lucy, and Krampitz, Sidney Diane. *Psychiatric Nursing.* 10th ed. F. A. Davis Company: Philadelphia, 1977.

Mereness, Dorothy A., and Taylor, Cecelia Monat. *Essentials of Psychiatric Nursing.* 10th ed. C. V. Mosbey Company: St. Louis, 1978.

Modly, Doris Matherny. "Paranoid States." *Journal of Psychiatric Nursing and Mental Health Services,* Vol. 16 No. 5 (May, 1978), 35-37.

Morgan, Arthur James, and Moreno, Judith Wilson. *The Practice of Mental Health Nursing: A Community Approach.* J. B. Lippincott Company: Philadelphia, 1973.

Nemiah, John C. *Foundations of Psychopathology.* Jason Aaronson, Inc.: New York, 1973.

Ostendorf, Mary. "Dan is Schizophrenic: Possible Causes, Probable Causes," *American Journal of Nursing,* Vol. 76 No. 6 (June, 1976), 944-947.

Price, Kenneth P. "Treating Psychosomatic Disorders With Behavior Therapy." *Nursing Digest,* Vol. 3 No. 6 (November/December, 1975), 12-19.

Provost, Judith. "Intervention in a Schizoaffective Depressive Behavior Pattern: a Behavioral Approach." *Perspectives in Psychiatric Care,* Vol. 12 No. 2 (1974), 86-89.

Roberts, Joanne M. "What is Loneliness?" *Perspectives in Psychiatric Care,* Vol. 10 No. 5 (1972), 227-231.

Rouslin, Sheila. "A Psychoanalytic View of Homosexuality: An Interview with Joseph J. Geller, M.D." *Perspectives Of Psychiatric Care,* Vol. 16 No. 2 (March/April, 1978), 76-79.

Rowe, Clarence J. *An Outline of Psychiatry.* 6th ed. Wm. C. Brown Company, Publishers: Dubuque, Iowa, 1975.

Salzman, Leon. *The Obsessive Personality.* Science House: New York, 1968.

Schmagin, Barbara G., and Pearlmutter, Deanna R. "The Pursuit of Unhappiness: The Secondary Gains of Depression." *Perspectives in Psychiatric Care,* Vol. 15 No. 2 (1977), 63-65.

Woodruff, Robert A., Jr.; Goodwin, Donald W.; and Guze, Samuel B. *Psychiatric Diagnosis.* Oxford University Press: New York, 1977.

Woodward, Carolyn Adams. "Wernicke-Korsakoff Syndrome: A Case Approach." *Journal of Psychiatric Nursing and Mental Health Services,* Vol. 16 No. 4 (April, 1978), 38-41.

part 3

chapter 15

nursing intervention for patients with thought disorders

learning objectives
> On completion of this chapter the reader should be able to:
>
> 1 Identify the four major areas of disruption in the thought process.
> 2 Distinguish between each of the identified problems.
> 3 Identify specific nursing interventions for each of the problem areas.
> 4 Understand the rationale on which each intervention is based.

The mind is a multisensory data bank of a million moments of "now." Thought is a functioning process of the brain that regulates the barometer of daily living experiences. It is the filtering and processing mechanism for the integration of inputs from the micro and macro environments. At the same time, the thought process is the output center of the brain; through speech, behavior and body language the thought process publicly announces the physical and emotional status of the individual to others.

This chapter is concerned with disturbances in the thought process. We identify four common patient problems requiring nursing intervention: disorientation, inability to follow directions, inability to focus on reality and illogical and unreasonable sequence of thought perception. The primary nursing care goal for patients with these problems is reorientation to reality.

disorientation

Disorientation is reflected by a disruption in the three spheres: the individual cannot recognize time, place or person. These disruptions can occur in one, two or all spheres, the latter most generally occurring in patients with organic brain syndromes. The disoriented patient experiences confusion and a distorted awareness of persons and things around him. This distortion frequently produces a corresponding feeling of fear or hostility within the patient. This is particularly true for those patients whose disorientation is accompanied by delusions or hallucinations stemming from paranoia and agitation. To promote and maintain a therapeutic atmosphere conducive to reorientation, the nurse should approach the patient in a calm, nonthreatening, composed manner. This approach is conveyed through control of facial expression and body posture. The nurse is careful that her expression does not mirror surprise, fear or laughter at any statement or set of behaviors exhibited by the patient. Instead, her attitude is one of assurance, hopefulness and helpfulness.

Specific interventions the nurse might consider using to deal with the problem of disorientation are included in Table 15-1. They are divided according to the three spheres of time, place and person.

TABLE 15-1
DISORIENTATION: INTERVENTION AND RATIONALE

TIME:

Intervention	Rationale
Make available to the patient a clock, a calendar, a daily newspaper and *current* magazines.	to establish continuous, consistent, ready feedback
Provide access to radio or television and evaluate the patient's interpretation of the broadcasted material.	to help the patient remain active and alert
Refer to specific dates times and events. For example: "Mr. Jones, it is noon—time for lunch." And "Mrs. Jones, it is two o'clock—time for you to take your pill."	to orient the patient to time sequences
Encourage staff, other patients and family members to talk about time-related activity.	to provide security, diminish anxiety and reinforce continuous time input
Provide access to and encourage patient's participation in current community or hospital activities and functions such as baseball or football games, a Christmas party, July 4th picnic or trips to restaurants or shopping centers.	to establish associations between time and activity and to prevent further deterioration and disorientation
Check frequently and know the whereabouts of the patient at all times.	to provide protection and safety for the patient
Maintain a consistent time schedule.	to provide a sense of security and to establish time reference points

TABLE 15-1 (continued)

Intervention	Rationale
Give the patient a copy of his daily schedule.	to increase his feeling of self-worth and to provide him with a frame of reference

PLACE

Intervention	Rationale
Tell the patient where he is: identify the hospital, ward and room number; repeat all information as needed.	to decrease anxiety, to increase awareness and to promote a feeling of security
Show the patient a picture of the hospital or supply the patient with hospital brochure.	to reinforce verbal statements regarding whereabouts
Have the patient explore and investigate his room and ward setting.	to maximize contact with reality through the use of sensory perception
Designate the patient's room with a nameplate on the door.	to decrease frustration and to provide a means of increasing independent functioning
Explain sounds the patient might hear, for example, the closing of the elevator door, carts being wheeled through the hall and the paging and ward intercommunication system.	to decrease fear responses and to prevent mounting levels of anxiety
Identify personnel by title: nurse, physician, nursing assistant	to establish points of reference in reality
Accompany the patient when he leaves the ward	to provide protection and safety for the patient

PERSON

Intervention	Rationale
Address the patient by name and title.	to re-establish and reinforce identity
Instruct staff, patients and visitors to address the patient by name.	to prevent confusion, to reinforce reality and to establish a pattern of consistency
Permit the patient to keep personal possessions such as clothes, books, pictures or significant mementoes.	to maintain a sense of personal identity in an atmosphere that is alien to the patient
Label clothing and possessions with the patient's name.	to establish a point of reference for the patient and to prevent others from encroaching on the patient's identity
Provide the patient with and encourage him to carry an identification card.	to provide a tangible means of identification
Explore with the patient his perception of self and reinforce reality when appropriate.	to correct misinterpretations and to provide consensual validation and feedback

inability to follow directions

The inability to follow directions manifests itself when an individual is confused, fearful, hostile, preoccupied or exhibits a faulty memory pattern. Thought disruption interferes with communication reception; thus, blockages and misinterpretations in the communicated message often occur. Because stimulus reception is decreased interpretations are often inaccurate. The patient will then show increased anxiety and will frequently express concern regarding these disturbances. Patients who frequently display the inability to follow directions are those who may be described as being depressed, psychotic, organic, or who have been hospitalized for a long period of time and are referred to as having institutional chronicity. Cultivation of an unhurried, patient, reassuring approach by the nurse along with the adoption of an attitude that is both positive and empathetic is perhaps the most effective basis for intervention needed to assist the patient in sorting out the real from the unreal.

Specific interventions for dealing with the inability to follow directions are shown in Table 15-2.

TABLE 15-2
INABILITY TO FOLLOW DIRECTIONS—INTERVENTION AND RATIONALE

Intervention	Rationale
Use simple, concrete terminology when talking with the patient.	to reduce the possibility of misinterpretation and confusion
Be direct.	to reduce the number of choices
Speak clearly in a quiet, well-modulated tone.	to decrease distortions and to promote a feeling of comfort
Repeat for the patient instructions or information as often as needed.	to insure that the patient has heard and understood and to decrease the patient's frustration
Ask the patient to restate instructions or information.	to correct misinterpretations immediately
Observe the patient's behavior.	to determine effectiveness of instructions
Remind and reorient the patient with respect to the usual daily routines.	to reduce confusion and to help the patient develop a pattern for daily living
Provide the patient with needed instructions immediately prior to any procedure or activity.	to decrease anxiety and to contribute toward the successful completion of the activity
Write out for the patient instructions or schedules.	to provide the patient with a handy reference
Encourage the patient to ask questions.	to assist the patient in clarification of thoughts
Label clearly and legibly such areas as the bathroom, the lounge, the physician's office and the patient's room.	to promote environmental awareness and a sense of security for the patient

TABLE 15-2 (continued)

Intervention	Rationale
Limit sensory input.	to decrease the amount of stimuli (distractors)
Limit choices.	to decrease frustration
Provide adequate lighting in halls, bathrooms, etc.	to prevent fear and to promote safety
Make frequent rounds at night.	to provide reassurance, comfort and safety
Make use of volunteers to sit with the patient when staff are not available.	to provide comfort, to promote a sense of security and to convey concern
Make sure areas such as the medication room or the cleaning and supply cupboards are inaccessible to the patient.	to promote safety for the patient
Make frequent, brief contacts with the patient throughout the day.	to maintain the patient's contact with reality
Provide a nightlight for the patient's room.	to provide safety and to reduce visual, environmental distortions

inability to focus on reality

The inability to focus on reality is encountered in those individuals who consistently and excessively rely on the use of such defensive operations as rationalization, denial and projection. This nursing care problem can also be identified in those individuals who manifest circumstantiality and flight of ideas in order to avoid the threat reality holds for them. Because this avoidance results in movement away from reality, the patient will usually display marked anxiety, distrust and fear of becoming involved. Other behavioral manifestations include suspiciousness of other people—their intent toward him and the accompanying fear of possible harm by them; distortions and/or exaggerations of what exists; isolation, agitation, hostility, anger and identity crises; and confused, incoherent speech patterns. The nurse should use an approach that is slow, deliberate and cautiously friendly. Her attitude should reflect subdued warmth, integrity and openmindedness. These attitudes are displayed through the presentation of the nurse as an individual who wishes to be helpful and to make known the facts, and who is willing to be available but does not force communication. Rather, the nurse, after assuming the initiative, steps back and waits for the patient to take the lead.

Specific interventions the nurse might adopt to facilitate the goal of reality reorientation for those patients who display an inability to focus on reality are shown in table 15-3.

TABLE 15-3
INABILITY TO FOCUS ON REALITY–INTERVENTION AND RATIONALE

Intervention	Rationale
Recognize and verbally express recognition to the patient of his loss of contact with reality.	to assure the patient that his problem is known and acknowledged by those providing care
Encourage the patient to be actively involved in his current activities.	to increase the patient's contact with reality and to decrease the fear of involvement with others
Demonstrate interest in the patient's physical well-being.	to establish trust and to indicate the nurse's concern
Redirect the patient's anger into appropriate channels such as work or recreational activities that require physical energy.	to promote socially acceptable behavior and to decrease the possibility of inappropriate acting out
Control the patient's environment with respect to: noise, lights, people and activities.	to decrease the environmental distractions which tend to stimulate inappropriate responses
Limit activity in which competition is a significant factor.	to reduce stress, anxiety, hostility and frustration
Provide simple tasks.	to allow for successful completion and so increase the patient's feeling of self-worth
Give merited recognition.	to build self-esteem and to increase trust and rapport toward the nurse
Maintain spatial distance between the nurse and the patient.	to promote comfort, to provide maneuvering room and to decrease anxiety
Keep promises.	to promote trust and to reduce fear
Be honest and open.	to facilitate communication and to promote trust
Supply needed facts.	to increase understanding and to prevent distortions and doubts
Invite, not demand, patient response.	to allow the patient to move at his own pace
Interrupt and refocus meaningless communication and purposeless activity.	to re-establish contact with reality
Present and discuss alternatives.	to assist the patient to find and use more effective methods of adaptation
Confront inappropriate and unacceptable behavior.	to help the patient to recognize the inappropriateness of his behavior
Ask the patient to make realistic commitments.	to help the patient assume responsibility for his behavior
Hold the patient accountable for fulfillment of commitments.	to maintain and reinforce reality expectations of responsible behavior

illogical and unreasonable sequence of thought perception

Illogical and unreasonable sequence of thought perception occurs within individuals who experience distorted or exaggerated sensory perception. These individuals are responding to the distorted or exaggerated sensory integration from within the unconscious mind. In addition, illogical and unreasonable thought perception also may be found in persons whose ideas tend to be rigid, repetitive and excessively personalized. Consequently, there is a marked decrease in the person's ability to communicate because of this rigidity, misinterpretation and personally subjective responses. The patient is able to verbalize but the meaning and intent of the message is not always readily apparent since its significance is known only to the patient. Because of the incoherent speech and lack of ability to be understood, the patient experiences frustration, anxiety, suspicion, rejection and isolation. In order to assist the patient in achieving contact with reality and decreased distortion, the nurse must understand the dynamics of thought disorders and approach the patient with persistent effort and consistent acceptance. The nurse must approach the patient in a nonthreatening manner and with the attitudes of advocacy and therapeutic involvement, such as in the examples outlined in Table 15-4.

TABLE 15-4
ILLOGICAL AND UNREASONABLE SEQUENCE OF THOUGHT PERCEPTION—
INTERVENTION AND RATIONALE

Intervention	Rationale
Initiate frequent, regular contacts with the patient.	to provide contact with reality and to promote trust
Remain with the patient despite silence, inappropriate behavior or ineffective communication.	to express unconditional acceptance, interest and concern
Remain expectant and focus attention on the patient.	to convey interest, attention and respect for the patient
Listen carefully to the patient.	to pick up cues from the patient that will assist the nurse in the decoding of messages
Pay attention to details and avoid speaking in generalities.	to reinforce reality by separating the real from the unreal
Verify interpretations.	to assist the patient in the use of consensual validation for the establishment of a reality orientation
Clarify patient's use of the generalized "they."	to make communication explicit
Identify and clarify with the patient differences between his thoughts, feelings and behavior.	to assist the patient in sorting out discrepancies in these areas

TABLE 15-4 (continued)

Intervention	Rationale
Tell the patient that his message is not understood or followed.	to act as a "sounding board" for reality feedback
Question illogical thinking.	to interrupt the progression of illogical thought and to reorient the patient to reality
Set limits on and openly discourage "crazy talk."	to discourage the patient's preoccupation with fantasy
Refrain from responding to the "crazy talk" as if the meaning were clearly understood.	to prevent falsification of reality
Refocus communication on the present.	to restore psychological equilibrium
Confront the patient with his thoughts and encourage him to make judgments regarding them.	to help the patient sort out the real from the unreal
Create situations in which the patient is likely to experience success.	to provide new, corrective satisfying experiences to replace negative attitudes about self
Respect requests.	to develop trust, convey respect and to maintain integrity
Prevent physiological and psychological overstimulation by such actions as temperature control, maintenance of nutrition and reduction in self-threat situations.	to provide comfort, safety and protection
Provide explanations for changes in daily routine.	to prevent hostility and to increase trust
Observe the patient and identify behavior which indicates specific pattern responses to illogical thinking.	to develop a base for planning effective intervention
Prevent and protect the patient from inaccurate sensory perceptions by such actions as the initiation of immediate contact with the patient, reduction of personal and environmental hazards and physical removal of the patient from the stress situation.	to provide safety, security, comfort and reduction in anxiety for the patient
Interrupt disturbed thinking process through the use of simple daily activities.	to maintain reality orientation and to decrease preoccupation with fantasy
Provide a time and place in which the patient may remain quiet and undisturbed.	to reduce environmental stress
Focus on the healthy aspects of the patient's personality.	to make use of the patient's assets in order to increase his functioning

The material presented in this chapter by no means encompasses all there is in the literature regarding patients who experience disturbances in the thought process. In fact, there is a myriad of literature dealing with crisis intervention and specific interventive techniques. This chapter does provide fundamental guidelines and rationales for the nurse to use in direct interventions with patients.

suggested readings

Arnold, Helen M. "Working with Schizophrenic Patients. Four A's: A Guide to One-to-One Relationships." *American Journal of Nursing*, Vol. 76 No. 6 (June, 1976), 941-943.

Clack, Janice. "An Interpersonal Technique for Handling Hallucinations." *Nursing Care of the Disoriented Patient.* American Nursing Association: New York, 1962, 16-26.

Cohen, Sidney, and Klein, Hazel K. "The Delirious Patient." *American Journal of Nursing*, Vol 58 No. 5 (May, 1958).

Cook, Judith. "Interpreting and Decoding Autistic Communication." *Perspectives in Psychiatric Care*, Vol. 9 No. 1 (1971), 24-29.

Dennehy, Ann. "Nursing Intervention in the Hallucinatory Process." *Exploring Progress in Psychiatric Nursing Practice.* American Nursing Association: New York, 1965, 22-25.

Donner, Gail. "The Treatment of A Delusional Patient." *American Journal of Nursing*, Vol. 69 No. 12 (December, 1969), 2642-2644.

Field, William. "When a Patient Hallucinates." *American Journal of Nursing*, Vol. 63 No. 2 (February, 1963), 80-81.

Field, William E., and Ruelke, Wylma. "Hallucinations and How To Deal With Them." *American Journal of Nursing*, Vol. 73 No. 4 (April, 1973), 638-640.

Frankel, Esther C. "I Spoke With the Dead." *American Journal of Nursing*, Vol. 69, No. 1 (January, 1969), 105-107.

Gerdes, Lenne. "The Confused or Delirious Patient." *American Journal of Nursing*, Vol. 68 No. 6 (June, 1968), 1228.

Lazaroff, Ura Ann Lantz. "The Prototaxic Mode of Experience: What is the Patient Trying to Tell You?" *Innovations in Nurse-Patient Relationships: Automatic or Reasoned Nurse Actions.* American Nursing Association: New York, 1962, 27-32.

Morris, Magdalena, and Rhodes, Martha. "Guidelines for the Care of Confused Patients." *American Journal of Nursing*, Vol. 72 No. 9 (September, 1972), 1630-1633.

Olson, Edith V. "The Nurse and Repersonalization of the Aged." *Effects of Stereotypes on Nursing Care.* American Nursing Association: New York, 1962, 28-34.

Schwartzman, Sylvia T. "The Hallucinating Patient and Nursing Intervention." *Journal of Psychiatric Nursing and Mental Health Services*, Vol. 13 No. 6 (November/December, 1976), 23-28, 33-36.

Travelbee, Joyce. *Intervention in Psychiatric Nursing.* F. A. Davis Co.: Philadelphia, 1970.

chapter 16

nursing intervention for patients with feeling disorders

learning objectives
On completion of this chapter the reader should be able to:

1 Identify the six major areas of disrupted feelings.
2 Distinguish between each of the identified feeling states.
3 Identify specific nursing interventions for each emotional state.
4 Understand the rationale on which each intervention is based.

Anxiety, fear, anger, loneliness, grief and pain are *real* and *human* feelings. They are an individual's response to crises, threats or seemingly uncontrollable situations. It is when these subjective responses become exaggerated, intensified or prolonged that they distort feelings. These distortions may occur for two reasons: as a result of the individual's inability to distinguish between the appropriateness or inappropriateness of the response; or as a result of the individual's growing dependence on the same response as a mode of adjustment or adaptation to *all* situations regardless of similarities or differences. Nursing intervention is directed toward relieving the intensity of the feeling through the provision of support, protection and education. The primary nursing care goal is *to sustain the patient during his period of discomfort while assisting him to learn new methods of adjustment.*

anxiety

Anxiety is a feeling state in which the individual experiences a pervasive, vague, intense sensation of apprehension or impending disaster that he feels cannot be prevented. Anxiety is caused either by threats to an individual's self-system or by threats to his biological integrity. This means that any situation which places the individual in jeopardy, either emotionally or physically, produces a feeling of "dis-ease" which, in turn, results in a concomitant disruption in the individual's ability to function. Because of the variations in the levels of anxiety experienced and because of its pervasiveness, the individual feels a wide range of subjective responses. These responses range from a generalized sensation of uncomfortableness to a state of panic. (See the section on anxiety in Chapter Eleven.) The most effective approach the nurse can assume in dealing with this type of distorted apprehension is one of thoughtful, calm objectivity. The nurse can best accomplish this approach through the expression of genuine concern for the patient and his well-being; by minimizing environmental stresses that may add to or increase the patient's level of anxiety; and by supporting and encouraging his ability to resolve the anxiety provoking issues together with her. This nursing intervention requires that the nurse's attitude convey to the patient her sense of his personal worth along with her advocacy and hopefulness.

Specific nursing interventions to deal with the problems of anxiety are listed in Table 16-1.

TABLE 16-1
ANXIETY—INTERVENTION AND RATIONALE

Intervention	Rationale
Acknowledge the pressure of anxiety.	to determine where the patient is and to identify what approach will serve in the best interest of the patient
Assess the level of anxiety.	to determine the degree of anxiety present and to determine the degree to which the patient's level of functioning is impaired
Recognize behavior patterns which indicate signs of mounting anxiety within the patient.	to establish a basis for the planning of individualized care and to prevent the anxiety from becoming more diffused
Identify and explore anxiety provoking issues.	to establish causations and to set priorities
Listen willingly.	to provide relief and to convey unqualified acceptance
Assist the patient to identify what he thought or felt prior to the onset of anxiety.	to help the patient to discover the cause of the triggering event
Discuss expectations and differences between expectations and outcomes.	to assist the patient to identify discrepancies between expectations and "real" outcomes

TABLE 16-1 (continued)

Intervention	Rationale
Explore details of similar experiences.	establish the sequence of events in the development of the patient's anxiety
Encourage the patient to identify his anxiety as anxiety.	to develop awareness in the patient
Explore what mechanisms, if any, produce relief.	to develop awareness and to evaluate effectiveness of the mechanism
Explore possible alternatives with the patient.	to identify successful coping mechanisms
Investigate somatic complaints: check vital signs, make physical assessments and report findings to the physician.	to rule out and *avoid* overlooking the possibility of the presence of physical illness and to maintain and strengthen the bond of trust between the nurse and the patient
Inform the patient of test results.	to maintain the nurse's integrity and to provide relief and reassurance for the patient
Deter the patient from dwelling on physical symptomology.	to provide the patient with relief by moving focus of attention from self and symptoms
Refrain from asking the patient *how* he feels.	to discourage dwelling on the problem
Provide patient with a full schedule of daily activities.	to involve the patient and thereby decrease the amount of time for introspection and obsessive preoccupation
Base activity program around old or known interests.	to prevent adding stress and to insure success
Provide suitable outlets for "working off" excess energy; cleaning the unit, running errands and assisting with routine activities.	to create a feeling of usefulness and to provide a means by which the nurse can give merited praise to strengthen the ego
Adhere to schedules and to patient's requests promptly.	to prevent anxiety from mounting and to convey the nurse's genuine concern
Stay with the patient when anxiety is mounting even if it means pacing the corridor with him.	to convey acceptance and to make use of any opportunity that might become available to reduce anxiety and to help the patient become more comfortable
Assess the patient's need for medication.	to provide relief from overwhelming anxiety

fear

Fear is an emotional response to an immediate, known and exaggerated, external, definite or perceived danger which produces within the individual a feeling of disequilibrium. This disequilibrium occurs because the individual is either unable or incapable of supplying the immediate demand response needed to deal with the danger. Fear may be either rational or irrational. It is always unpleasant, restrictive and it produces disorganized behavior. Therefore, to assist the patient toward restoration of equilibrium, the nurse should approach the patient with quiet, positive objectivity and self-confidence using the therapeutic self. In addition, the nurse needs to support the patient's own coping and problem solving mechanisms. The attitudes most needed by the nurse to make this intervention operational are those of open-mindedness and assurance.

Specific interventions designed to deal with the problem of fear are listed in Table 16-2.

TABLE 16-2
FEAR—INTERVENTION AND RATIONALE

Intervention	Rationale
Remain with the patient when he is verbally expressing fear or displaying fear response behavior.	to provide protection and support
Encourage the patient to express his awareness of danger.	to increase the patient's recognition and to establish causation
Reconstruct with the patient previously identified fear producing situations.	to establish causes, sequence and responses
Examine with the patient his responses to the stated danger.	to determine effectiveness of responses
Support and encourage the patient to vary his responses to the identified danger.	to assist the patient to discover effective adjustment techniques which reduce fear
Reduce or minimize identified environmental threats which produce fear; for example, if the patient expresses fear of people, assign him to a private room; assign the same staff member to provide nursing care and introduce new people one at a time.	to provide protection and support and to allow for adaptation and adjustment
Keep anxiety producing situations to a minimum: proceed slowly, reduce the number of choices and avoid confrontations.	to prevent the transformation of anxiety into fear
Focus a portion of each interaction on areas of capability rather than on areas of dysfunction.	to maximize the patient's assets and to create an atmosphere of acceptance
Give concrete assistance in the management of everyday affairs that tend to be fear producing such as budget planning, job hunting or child caring.	to demonstrate tangible evidence of the nurse's interest in providing immediate relief and to allow the patient freedom to work on more abstract or general problems

TABLE 16-2 (continued)

Intervention	Rationale
Promote relaxation through environmental and interpersonal means such as using soft lights and music, avoiding surprises and speaking in quiet tones.	to reduce fear provoking environmental and interpersonal stimuli and to provide soothing stimuli
Expose the patient gradually to any fear stimulus.	to desensitize the patient to fear stimuli and to promote successful adaptive responses

anger

Anger is a disruptive emotion indicative of displeasure, frustration and conflict. It is a compensatory response used by the individual to prevent feelings of utter helplessness and hopelessness from becoming overwhelming. Anger occurs when the individual feels he has failed in the attempt to meet the overpowering need to exert control over himself, situations, objects or others within his immediate environment. As a result of this presumed failure the individual perceives no other alternative open to him that will permit the maintenance of his independence and self-respect or ward off unpleasant outcomes except to become angry. Because of the need to control, the individual is likely to display a wide range of angry behaviors. Examples of behavior within this range are: irritation or procrastination; verbal threats or name calling; eruption of violence in the form of striking out; and the development of pathophysiology in the form of ulcerative colitis. To assist the individual to recognize his anger, identify its cause and develop successful methods of dissipation, the nurse must respect the physical space needed by the patient during the crisis. She must approach the patient in a nonthreatening, nonjudgmental and calmly confident manner. The most helpful attitudes the nurse needs to adopt in working with patients who are displaying anger are those of integrity and personal worth.

Specific interventions the nurse can employ in the nursing management of angry patients are listed in Table 16-3.

TABLE 16-3
ANGER—INTERVENTION AND RATIONALE

Intervention	Rationale
Observe the patient's behavior for signs of anger.	to identify and assess the patient and to safeguard the patient through early recognition and intervention
Ask direct questions relating to observations, such as: "Are you angry?" and, "Do you feel angry?"	to provide validation for observations and to assist the patient to recognize the presence of anger

TABLE 16-3 (continued)

Intervention	Rationale
Rephrase question if patient denies or represses, for example: "You look upset," and, "You sound distressed."	to clarify and verify observations regarding behavior and to facilitate recognition of anger
Focus the patient's communication on a description of his feelings, such as: "What do you mean when you say you are sad?" and, "Tell me more about being disappointed . . . frustrated . . . depressed."	to encourage expression of feelings and to prevent avoidance or denial of felt anger
Explore with the patient feelings associated with the anger, such as guilt, humiliation, dependency and fear.	to elicit the emotional recognition and acceptance of anger
Identify causative factors.	to assist the patient to understand the reason for his anger
Determine with the patient if the cause is realistic.	to evaluate the legitimacy of the anger
Explore with the patient his methods of dealing with anger.	to assist the patient in making a connection between the expressed feeling and the displayed behavior
Explore with the patient alternatives that are interpersonally and socially acceptable, for example, ask, "What could you do when the nurse keeps you waiting for your medications causing you to be late for your appointment with the doctor?"	to assist the patient in using the problem solving approach to develop an acceptable means of dealing with legitimate anger
Provide socially acceptable activities for the displacement of energy associated with angry feelings, such as physical exercise, weaving, typing and playing the piano.	to channel the expression of anger constructively, to foster feelings of accomplishment and to increase self-worth
Maintain your "cool" by refraining from resorting to retaliatory behavior.	to preserve integrity for the patient and the nurse and to prevent the situation from getting out of control
Allow the patient a "cooling down" period before exploring precipitating factors.	to assist in the development of control
Intervene and separate those patients who are mutually antagonistic.	to set limits and to provide a safe, comfortable environment
Set positive expectations and explain rules and regulations.	to forestall the development of or the increase in intensity of the anger
Hold the patient accountable for destructive acts.	to assist the patient in the development of responsible behavior
Meet requests, complaints and demands with thoughtfulness, respect and openmindedness.	to demonstrate acceptance of the patient, to provide an avenue for reasonability and to support the patient's feelings of self-worth

TABLE 16-3 (continued)

Intervention	Rationale
Provide external controls until such time as the patient is able to exercise self-control by: providing a quiet room, administering medication, removing harmful objects from the environment or using physical restraint.	to reduce the amount of tension experienced by the patient, to eliminate threats, to promote safety and to provide protection for the patient

loneliness

Loneliness is a severe, painful subjective state in which the individual feels that he does not belong and that no one cares. Loneliness is a symptom that usually compounds other psychiatric problems such as depression, some forms of psychoses, adjustment reactions and some transient situational disorders. The lonely individual perceives himself as being deprived of intimate relationships with other human beings and of the opportunity to share his thoughts, feelings, achievements and life with significant others. Because of the perceived deficit of intimacy in relationships, the patient experiencing loneliness often underestimates his abilities, underrates his achievements and loses the motivation necessary to solve problems. The lonely individual is unable to experience love; therefore, communication and sharing are dramatically decreased in turn inhibiting the development of therapeutic rapport. This individual's adjustment to life is marked by feelings of depression, dejection, despair and desolation. The behavior he displays reveals an almost total lack of caring for self and others. Some specific behaviors that indicate this lack include moodiness, self-deprecating acts, morbid preoccupation with death, suicidal ruminations or gestures and complete social isolation and withdrawal into a world of fantasy. In developing a therapeutic environment for the patient displaying the problem of loneliness, it is imperative that the nurse's approach be one that actively seeks out the patient, demonstrates genuine warmth and reflects loving concern. The attitudes the nurse cultivates to achieve this approach are those of hopefulness and involvement.

Specific nursing interventions for effectively dealing with the problem of loneliness are listed in Table 16-4.

TABLE 16-4
LONELINESS—INTERVENTION AND RATIONALE

Intervention	Rationale
Seek out the patient and spend time with him on a regularly scheduled basis.	to demonstrate concern and to let the patient know that he is not alone—he can rely on you

TABLE 16-4 (continued)

Intervention	Rationale
Discuss loneliness with the patient.	to determine what loneliness means to the patient and how he experiences it
Plan a regular schedule for the patient.	to prevent social isolation and to maintain contact with reality
Expect attendance and involvement at scheduled activities.	to create within the individual the idea that motivation comes from within the self
Discuss with the patient his feelings regarding involvement in activity.	to determine his level of involvement and its effectiveness in alleviating loneliness and to provide an opportunity to reinforce belonging and selfworth
Encourage involvement in group activities.	to foster a sense of belonging and identity
Acknowledge the patient's feeling of loneliness.	to convey empathy and understanding
Respond to request immediately— avoid delays.	to prevent interpretation of delay as rejection and proof of the patient's worthlessness
Reinforce the patient's identity by addressing him by name or by personally inviting him to attend the church service of his choice.	to maintain contact with reality and to establish feelings of personal worth
Touch the patient—pat him on the shoulder, lay a hand on his wrist or arm.	to indicate presence and to convey a feeling of genuine warmth and a sense of sharing
Assign the patient to useful, important tasks, for example: passing out lunch trays, helping sort clean laundry, taking responsibility for the care of the ward plants or pets.	to instill a sense of usefulness and productivity and to provide a basis for legitimate praise
Give merited praise.	to provide recognition for the successful completion of activities
Select occupational or recreational activities which are familiar to the patient and at which he is known to be successful.	to limit the possibility of failure and to provide an avenue for social intercourse
Encourage the patient to ventilate his feelings.	to relieve tension and to foster selfworth through acceptance
Focus the patient's communication on the present and the future.	to keep the patient oriented to reality and to prevent preoccupation with past problems
Encourage the patient to be socially assertive, that is, to develop and broaden his sphere of social activity.	to develop a sense of success in social communication, sharing and intimacy.

grief

Grief is an emotional state experienced by the individual following severe loss or prolonged deprivation. It occurs when an individual experiences the loss of a person, treasured object or part of the physical self. In grief there is a loss of love, a marked decrease in the sense of being needed, a feeling of abandonment and a decrease in the level of self-esteem and self-worth.

The behavioral science literature is increasingly enlightening on the processes of grief and mourning. Grief is complicated by guilt and depression, therefore, it is essential to the interventive technique to understand that guilt and depression are not the primary diagnoses. When the individual is suffering from severe loss or prolonged deprivation he generally seeks to deny the causes or to minimize the effect they have on him so that he will not have to deal with the resultant emotional issues.

The subjective experiences associated with grief can be described as existing on a continuum. It begins with the socially accepted "normal grief behavior" following the loss of a loved one, such as crying, frequent forgetfulness or temporary loss of time spans, and proceeds toward a severe, overpowering depression that can become pathologic in its manifestations, such as suicidal attempts, becoming reclusive, increasing malfunctioning on the job and even loss of contact with reality. In her practice the nurse may encounter the entire spectrum of the grief and mourning continuum, but it is only when the individual has become so overwhelmed that the nurse is requested, or deems it necessary to intervene on behalf of the patient.

The approach the nurse will find most effective in dealing with grief and mourning is one which is calm, objective, unhurried, flexible and consistent. She must acknowledge and recognize the significance the lost person, object or part of the self has for the individual and the system of interdependent functioning upon these objects the individual had as a part of his personally integrated framework of functioning. The attitudes needed to implement intervention and this approach are those of genuine concern, empathy, advocacy and hopefulness.

Specific interventions the nurse can employ to deal with the problem of grief are listed in Table 16-5.

TABLE 16-5
GRIEF—INTERVENTION AND RATIONALE

Intervention	Rationale
Organize and plan a schedule for the patient until the patient displays an ability to take over the planning and organizing process.	to meet the dependency needs of the patient
Consult the patient about the plans.	to encourage involvement
Encourage the patient to participate in activities of daily living.	to maintain contact with reality and to prevent regression

TABLE 16-5 (continued)

Intervention	Rationale
Limit available choices.	to reduce stress
Give directions and instructions and repeat as necessary.	to surmount the communication barrier produced by decreased perceptual awareness
Encourage the patient to verbalize feelings associated with loss.	to assist the patient in developing an awareness of predominant feelings
Discuss feelings of ambivalence, disappointment, resentment or anger.	to promote the patient's understanding of self
Remain with the patient despite his lack of ability to verbalize.	to demonstrate to the patient unconditional acceptance
Break silence periodically with positive, nonthreatening statements of fact, such as: "Five minutes have gone by, I will be with you for fifteen more minutes" or "I'll be here tomorrow."	to establish a sense of "thereness" and "relatedness" with the patient
Allow time for responses when communicating with the patient.	to accomodate the patient's distortions in perception and delayed response time
Listen patiently to repititious verbalizations of guilt or self-blame.	to demonstrate to the patient nonjudgmental acceptance
Interrupt monologues and refocus on feelings.	to penetrate the defensive shield of superficial communication
Remain with the patient during nonverbal ventilation of feelings such as crying, sobbing, screaming and introspective staring.	to offer empathetic support to the patient
Assist the patient to find meaning in his loss through his personal framework of philosophy and value systems.	to offer support, encouragement and hope
Provide an opportunity for visitation from the clergy.	to sustain the patient in his religious beliefs and to enable him to grow spiritually
Give special attention to physical needs: oral hygiene, physical cleanliness, appropriate dress and general attractiveness in appearance.	to demonstrate care and concern of the nurse, to prevent halitosis, to stimulate taste buds, to encourage appetite, to insure protection against climactic changes, to promote self-concept and to encourage general physical well-being of the patient
Provide a balanced diet of frequent, small feedings, and assist with eating by giving verbal encouragement to eat, cutting up food or feeding the patient.	to meet the nutritional needs of the patient and to prevent weight loss
Make meal times an attractive and pleasurable experience by determining likes and dislikes, having relatives bring	to stimulate appetite, to promote socialization and to increase feelings of self-worth

TABLE 16-5 (continued)

Intervention	Rationale
favorite foods from home, adding warm, bright colors to place settings and sitting with the patient while he is eating.	
Provide physical exercise.	to maintain the patient's normal physiological processes such as circulation, elimination and nutrition
Promote rest and sleep by providing warm milk or a hot tub at bed time, remaining with the patient until he is asleep, checking periodically for wakefulness and remaining with the patient to determine the cause of sleeplessness or to administer prescribed hypnotics.	to prevent loss of rest and to promote the patient's physical and emotional comfort
Assign small repetitive tasks.	to relieve feelings of guilt
Observe for clues indicative of suicidal behavior such as verbal statements in which the patient says "good-bye" instead of "good night"; or when the patient indicates that everything will be fine tomorrow.	to safeguard the patient from self-destructive behavior
Alert *all* staff members to suicide potential.	to decrease potential of environmental hazards and to provide safety and security for the patient

pain

Pain is an emotional phenomena of the mind, and, as such, it is a highly individualized subjective experience. Pain is *real*. Pain is *hurt*. And pain is suffering, anguish and agony. It can be experienced emotionally, physically, psychologically and spiritually. There is dull pain, excruciating pain, throbbing pain, tormenting pain, searing pain, and the pain associated with embarrassment, as in a social faux pas. The list of adjectives used to describe pain and its intensity are almost endless. But words can hardly capture the true substance of pain for, unlike emotional states, pain is undeniably a particularly unique and individualized sensation. What one individual may experience as painful may not be painful for another. Each individual's threshold of pain varies based on his philosophical framework, value system, and/or his interpretations regarding the cause of pain. Thus pain is valued, feared, accepted, denied or fought. An individual can interpret a painful experience as a challenge, as a punishment, as an enemy, as a warning or as a learning experience. The nurse's approach should be one of sympathetic, empathetic personal warmth. The attitudes needed by the nurse to carry out this intervention are those of empathy, genuine concern and sympathy.

Specific interventions the nurse can use to deal with the problem of pain are listed in Table 16-6.

TABLE 16-6
PAIN—INTERVENTION AND RATIONALE

Intervention	Rationale
Pay close attention to what the patient says about his pain with respect to site, frequency, type, duration, possible cause, contributing factors and feelings prior to the onset of discomfort.	to obtain a basis for intervention and to demonstrate interest and concern for the patient's well-being
Observe body posture and positioning during pain episodes.	to determine pain reaction and the effectiveness of the patient's coping mechanisms
Explore with the patient those measures he has used in the past to reduce painful sensations.	to identify the patient's coping mechanisms and to support and encourage his use of effective comfort devices
Administer medication before pain increases in intensity and becomes unbearable.	to decrease actual pain perception and promote comfort
Maintain optimum environmental conditions by decreasing the level of noise, eliminating unpleasant odors, dimming glaring lights and maintaining even temperature and air flow.	to promote comfort and to prevent possible intensification of pain
Exercise care in changing the patient's position, making his bed and handling equipment on or near him.	to prevent jarring the patient and causing increased pain
Listen attentively to the patient's expression of feelings.	to demonstrate the nurse's sympathetic and empathetic concern and understanding of the patient and to alleviate distress
Report signs and symptoms of discomfort immediately.	to share information for the purpose of providing the patient with relief
Refocus patient's attention away from self and the pain.	to decrease pain perception, to increase level of tolerance and to promote comfort
Accept the patient's verbalizations regarding the intensity of the painful experience.	to establish rapport and foster trust and to expedite implementation of alternative coping mechanisms
Explore the meaning of pain to the patient from a physical, psychological, social and spiritual viewpoint.	to increase the nurse's awareness, understanding and acceptance of the patient and to support his endeavors to find meaning in his suffering

In this chapter we have presented six of the most universal and significant human feelings that are most likely to be subjected to distortion. These human feelings are those which the nurse will most frequently encounter in her daily practice, whether the practice is within the setting of a psychiatric facility, an outpatient clinic or a medical-surgical unit of a general hospital. Because of the constant need to deal with these problems it is essential that the nurse identify, acknowledge and understand the spectrum of anxiety, fear, anger, loneliness, grief and pain as they move from the accepted and tolerable norm to the severe and traumatizing level of pathology. It is only within the context of knowledge complemented by empathy, understanding, care and concern that the nurse can make effective therapeutic interventions on behalf of the patient.

suggested readings

Bier, Ruth. "Motivation of the Chronically Ill Aged Patient." *Culture, Atmosphere and Social Organization: Effects On Nursing Care of the Patients.* American Nursing Association: New York, 1962, 34-39.

Burd, Shirley F., and Marshall, Margaret A., eds. *Some Clinical Approaches to Psychiatric Nursing.* Macmillan Co.: New York, 1963.

Burnside, Irene. "Touching is Talking." *American Journal of Nursing*, Vol. 73 No. 12 (December, 1973), 2060.

Carter, Elizabeth W. "A Proposed Technique of Nursing Intervention With Patients Who Deny Mental Illness." *Nursing Approaches to Denial of Illness.* American Nursing Association: New York, 1962, 38-44.

Engle, George. "Grief and Grieving." *American Journal of Nursing*, Vol. 64 No. 9 (September, 1964), 93-98.

Epstein, Charlotte. *Nursing the Dying Patient.* Reston Publishing Co., Inc.: Reston, Virginia, 1975.

Hashizume, Sato. "She Asked: Am I Going Crazy?" *Nursing '75,* Vol. 5 No. 2 (February, 1975), 12-15.

Hauser, Marilyn Jean, and Feinberg, Doris R. "An Operational Approach to the Delayed Grief and Mourning Process." *Journal of Psychiatric Nursing and Mental Health Services*, Vol. 14 No. 7 (July, 1976), 29-35.

Irving, Susan. *Basic Psychiatric Nursing.* W. B. Saunders Co.: Philadelphia, 1973.

Kaufmann, Margaret A., and Brown, Dorothy E. "Pain Wears Many Faces." *American Journal of Nursing*, Vol. 61 No. 1 (January, 1961), 48-51.

Kavanaugh, Robert L. "Dealing Naturally With the Dying." *Nursing '76*, Vol. 6 No. 10 (October, 1976), 23-29.

Koch, Joanne. "When Children Meet Death." *Psychology Today* (August, 1977), 64-67.

Luckman, Joan, and Sarenson, Karen. "What Patient's Actions Tell You About Their Feelings, Fears and Needs." *Nursing '75*, Vol. 5 No. 2 (February, 1975), 54-61.

McCaffrey, Margo. "Patients in Pain." *Nursing '75*, Vol. 3 No. 6 (June, 1973), 41-50.

Mereness, Dorothy, and Taylor, Cecelia Monat. *Essentials of Psychiatric Nursing.* 10th ed. C. V. Mosbey Co.: St. Louis, 1978.

Moustakas, Clark E. *Portraits of Loneliness and Love.* Prentice-Hall, Inc.: Englewood Cliffs, New Jersey, 1974.

Newsome, Betty H., and Oden, Gloria. "Nursing Intervention in Panic." *Emergency Intervention by the Nurse*, American Nursing Association: New York, 1962, 15-21.

Neylan, Margaret Prowse. "The Depressed Patient." *American Journal of Nursing*, Vol. 61 No. 7 (July, 1961), 77-78.

Papoff, David. "Probe—What Are Your Feelings About Death and Dying?" *Nursing '75*, Vol. 5 No. 8 (August, 1975), 15-24.

Preddy, Erica. "Leave Me Alone." *Nursing '75*, Vol. 5 No. 1 (January, 1975), 13-15.

Preston, Tonie. "When Words Fail." *American Journal of Nursing*, Vol. 73 No. 12 (December, 1973), 2064-2066.

Smiley, Dorothy M. "Nursing the Patient Who is Experiencing Chronic Pain." *Nursing of Patients With Loss of Perceptions.* American Nurses Association: New York, 1962, 23-29.

Strauss, Anselm; Fagerhaugh, Shizuko Y.; and Glaser, Lorney. "Pain—An Organizational–Work–Interactional Perspective." *Nursing Outlook,* Vol. 22 No. 9 (September, 1974), 560-566.

Swanson, Ardis R. "Communicating With Depressed Persons." *Perspectives in Psychiatric Care*, Vol. 13 No. 2 (1975), 63-67.

Thomas, Mary D.; Baker, Joan M.; and Estes, Nada J. "Anger? A Tool For Developing Self-Awareness." *American Journal of Nursing,* Vol. 70, No. 12 (December, 1970), 2586-2590.

Thompson, Linda. "Sensory Deprivation: A Personal Experience." *American Journal of Nursing*, Vol. 73 No. 2 (February, 1973), 266-268.

Westercamp, Twilla M. "Suicide." *American Journal of Nursing*, Vol. 75 No. 2 (February, 1975), 260-262.

Wiggins, Jack G., and Henderson, Robert W. *Coping with Personal Depression.* Berea, Ohio: Personal Growth Press, 1968.

Williams, Jane C. "Understanding The Feelings of the Dying." *Nursing '76*, Vol. 6 No. 3 (March, 1976), 52-56.

Zahourek, Rothlyn and Jensen, Joseph S. "Grieving and the Loss of the Newborn." *American Journal of Nursing*, Vol. 73 No. 5 (May, 1973), 836-839.

chapter 17

nursing intervention for patients with disturbances in behavior

learning objectives

On completion of this chapter, the reader should be able to:

1 Identify, define and describe these behaviors: negativistic, regressive, aggressive, manipulative, self-destructive, hyperactive, compulsive, suspicious.

2 Identify the interventions necessary for each of the eight behavior categories.

3 Understand the rationale for each of the interventive techniques.

In the practice of psychiatric-mental health nursing, the nurse encounters many forms of behavior associated with psychiatric disorders, emotional disturbances, stress, crisis and conflict. These behaviors differ both in mode and degree according to the patient, his circumstances, life experiences and his life style. In addition, we cannot overlook the influences of culture, environment and family history which may contribute to and influence the patient's system of belief and coping devices. All these factors when taken together lead themselves to the development of individualized pathological behavioral manifestations.

Of no small consequence, therefore, is the fact that nursing staff in institutional or hospital settings are consistently being confronted with a spectrum of behaviors that are classified vaguely as "management problems." Thus, it is vital that the nurse learn about and understand the dynamics of such behaviors; learn and be able to employ methods of appropriate and successful interventions and understand the rationale behind the use of such interventive techniques. Such knowledge creates the best ambiance for the therapeutic community, minimizes friction between patients of varying personalities and maximizes the ultilization of professional staff time toward the treatment of the whole patient.

We identify eight major, common disturbances in behavior. They are: negativistic, regressive, aggressive, manipulative, self-destructive, hyperactive, compulsive and suspicious. The primary nursing care goal for patients experiencing behavioral disturbances is to *bring about a change in behavior.*

negativistic behavior

Negativistic behavior is resistance. It is conveyed through actions which are in opposition to general expectations. The individual demonstrates an inability to comply. This inability is displayed through such behavioral actions and attitudes as procrastination, passivity, silence, blatant refusal, avoidance and denial. To meet the needs of a patient displaying negativistic behavior the nurse should adopt a calm, consistent, accepting, nonjudgmental, nonpunitive approach. The attitudes the nurse must cultivate in order to carry out this type of approach are those of openmindedness, hopefulness and understanding the dynamics of negativistic behavior.

Specific nursing interventions directed toward dealing with the problem of negativistic behavior are listed in Table 17-1.

TABLE 17-1
NEGATIVISTIC BEHAVIOR—INTERVENTION AND RATIONALE

Interventions	Rationale
Present and explain expectations.	to set realistic goals and to limit the direction negative behavior can take
Eliminate the possibility of negative choices; for example, since the expectation is that the patient will attend occupational therapy, the choices presented to the patient are for him either to attend alone or to be escorted by a member of the staff.	to discourage negative responses, to encourage the development of responsible behavior and to prevent deterioration or loss of essential behaviors necessary for living
Identify with the patient the manner in which he expresses negativistic behavior.	to establish the patient's awareness of behaviors requiring change
Identify positive reinforcers.	to determine what rewards to select for the patient in order to make the behavioral change contract effective

TABLE 17-1 (continued)

Intervention	Rationale
Draw up a behavioral change contract with the patient including a daily activity schedule; a list of behaviors to be changed; choices allowed, if any; rewards for fulfilling contracted expectations and penalties for default.	to clearly identify for the patient staff expectations, to verbally reinforce positive responses and to encourage self-motivation
Present patient and all concerned staff with a copy of the contract.	to act as a positive reminder for the patient and to promote consistency of approach among staff
Coordinate all staff efforts on behalf of the patient.	to promote a unified approach and to reinforce consistent application of the contract
Inform and elicit support of significant others who relate to the patient.	to provide consistency, to assist concerned others to develop understanding of the patient and an awareness of the treatment program and to promote acceptance of the patient
Closely monitor the patient's progress.	to assess the degree to which the patient is involved, to evaluate the effectiveness of the contract and to establish a data base for further intervention
Record observations accurately.	to facilitate the process
Re-assess and evaluate the contract periodically with patient and staff.	to determine progress and basis for renegotiation of contract
Renegotiate contract as needed.	to provide care and treatment according to patient's needs and progress
Effect consistent, persistent approaches to the patient.	to demonstrate acceptance, establish rapport, build trust and increase the patient's feeling of security
Assist the patient to verbalize feelings about his negativistic behavior; for example, if the patient refuses to participate in a routine daily activity, say, "You seem to resent having to make your bed today"; if the patient is silent during interactions, say, "Perhaps there is something which is difficult for you to discuss."	to indicate to the patient the nurse's interest and concern as to why he is behaving as he does, and to interrupt negative behavior patterns

regressive behavior

Regressive behavior is a selective, defensive operation in which the individual resorts to earlier, childish, labile, less complex patterns of behavior. These behaviors were often prevalent and even considered appropriate during childhood; however, when the adult behaves this way, he is considered maladapted. Regressive behavior seldom permeates all areas of an individual's personality structure; even the most severely regressed patient retains some potential for the development of adequate coping devices necessary for the maintenance of survival. Some examples of regressive behavior which illustrate the extent to which the individual can be incapacitated are egocentricity or preoccupation with self, tantrums, pouting, refusal to communicate or to participate in the ordinary activities of daily living, daydreams, hallucinations, delusions, isolation or the assumption of a fetal position. The type of nursing approach needed to care for individuals with regressive behavior is one that is warm, persistent, patient and nonthreatening. To achieve this approach the nurse's attitude must be one of personal worth, involvement and hopefulness.

Specific nursing interventions used to deal with regressive behavior are listed in Table 17-2.

TABLE 17-2
REGRESSIVE BEHAVIOR—INTERVENTION AND RATIONALE

Intervention	Rationale
Initiate short, frequent contacts with the patient.	to convey the nurse's interest and concern and to emphasize to the patient the nurse's attitude that the patient has personal worth
Remain with the patient for designated periods of time.	to establish rapport and trust
Maintain the nurse's focus of attention on the patient during periods of contact: look at the patient; address him by name; and direct communication specifically toward him.	to re-emphasize personal worth
Use simple language and specific words.	to prevent misunderstanding and misinterpretation of reality
Use short sentences.	to promote better understanding of the communicated messages
Speak quietly, distinctly, and directly to the patient.	to decrease potential anxiety and to prevent loss of interest and understanding due to the patient's limited attention span
Be honest and open with the patient; for example, keep promises; provide necessary information; give easy-to-follow directions and explanations for procedures.	to establish trust, to facilitate communication and to offer him a reassuring, anxiety-free interpersonal contact
Give merited praise and recognition based on specific, accurate observations such as, "I see you're wearing your new dress today" and, "You made	to help the patient to rebuild his self-esteem

TABLE 17-2 (continued)

Intervention	Rationale
your bed already" and, "You finished your project in O.T."	
Allow the patient to be as dependent as he needs to be; for example, if patient is mute, encourage him but don't demand a verbal response; if patient refuses to eat, prepare and serve food attractively, encourage and assist with food intake, feed if necessary; if the patient is incontinent, provide clean clothes, bedding and institute a toileting schedule.	to meet dependency needs and guard against excessive anxiety and reinforcing feelings of rejection or subjection while preventing further ego disintegration and to maintain a nonjudgmental, nonpunitive approach
Observe the patient for signs and symptoms of physical illness.	to promote health and prevent illness
Allow the patient sufficient time to respond.	to demonstrate the nurse's willingness to proceed at the patient's own pace
Encourage the patient to gradually assume initiative.	to assist the patient to move toward reality
Gradually increase the complexity and scope of the patient's decision making.	to reinforce reality and to encourage responsible, independent functioning
Gradually increase exposure to people and environmental changes.	to keep the level of anxiety to a minimum
Introduce the patient to simple, routine, familiar activities.	to reach out to the patient and to reintroduce reality in a nonthreatening and potentially anxiety-free atmosphere
Encourage and assist the patient to carry out activities.	to increase self-esteem, to reinforce the bond of trust, and to use the activity as a focus for interpersonal communication
Plan and initiate an uncomplicated, structured daily routine.	to provide a basis for maintaining contact with reality
Deal with the patient on an adult level—avoid nicknames, slang, street language or crude language.	to demonstrate respect, to increase self-esteem and to convey a sense of personal worth
Control environmental conditions such as lighting, temperature, noise and contacts with other people.	to provide the correct amount of stimuli needed by the patient and to prevent him from becoming dominated by the environment, that is, from becoming institutionalized
Foster realism in daily living by having the patient wear his own personal clothing, eat with the proper utensils and by promoting conversation in the dining room.	to increase contact with reality, to promote socially acceptable behavior and to increase socialization
Observe the patient for behavior pattern responses to environmental, interpersonal and intrapsychic situations.	to gather information for planning future interventions and to increase knowledge about and understanding of the patient

TABLE 17-2 (continued)

Intervention	Rationale
Recognize mounting tensions based on known behavioral responses.	to facilitate the planning of successful intervention on behalf of the patient
Intervene before regression becomes more rigid or severe.	to interrupt the regressive pattern and refocus the patient on reality
Accept the patient's need to test the nurse's integrity, reliability, care, concern and degree of involvement.	to foster trust, develop rapport and increase the patient's self concept
Identify "testing measures" used by the patient.	to increase knowledge and understanding about the patient
Recognize situations in which "testing" is prevalent.	to plan intervention
Respond to the patient who is testing by acknowledgment and confrontation, a search for causation and a re-evaluation of the approach to the patient.	to reinforce reality, and promote realistic security operations and to set limits on unacceptable behavior

aggressive behavior

Aggressive behavior is forceful self-assertion which tends to be destructive in nature. Aggressive behavior is attack behavior which evokes retaliatory or defensive responses. The individual resorts to aggressive behavior when he perceives there is no other form of adaptation available to him when exposed to excessive stimulation. The patient displaying aggressive behavior is hypersensitive, resentful and believes that he is subjected to control and domination by circumstances or people. The overriding emotional response is anger that is discharged openly and directly or subtly and indirectly toward the physical or interpersonal environment. The kind of therapeutic atmosphere needed by patients who display aggressive behavior is one in which the nurse takes a calm, quiet, structured, accepting approach. To create such an atmosphere the nurse must cultivate the attitudes of openmindedness, integrity, temperate firmness and patience.

Specific nursing interventions the nurse can use to deal with aggressive behavior are listed in Table 17-3

TABLE 17-3
AGGRESSIVE BEHAVIOR—INTERVENTION AND RATIONALE

Intervention	Rationale
Initiate frequent, regularly scheduled contacts.	to demonstrate the nurse's acceptance of the patient regardless of his behavior
Maintain spatial distance between self and patient.	to prevent the patient from feeling over-powered or dominated by the presence of "authority"

TABLE 17-3 (continued)

Intervention	Rationale
Provide clear, concise explanations for all rules and regulations.	to set control through definition of limits and to set positive expectations for responsible behavior
Use a positive approach—make suggestions rather than give commands; invite participation rather than make demands; redirect action rather than imposing external controls.	to foster the building of trust and to emphasize integrity and reliability of the nurse
Be honest and open in communications.	to reduce fear, anxiety and to lessen the patient's sense of domination and helplessness
Remain rational and dependable.	to convey the nurse's sincerity and security, thus promoting the patient's feeling of security and trust in the nurse and to avoid power struggles
Listen to complaints and attempt to identify their legitimacy.	to give recognition to the patient in order to increase his sense of integrity
Respond positively to reasonable demands and requests.	to re-emphasize the patient's sense of personal worth and minimize the patient's potential loss of control
Absorb verbal expressions of anger, resentment, bitterness, belittling or sarcasm.	to demonstrate acceptance of the individual regardless of behavior
Define with the patient the extent of the problem.	to convey the nurse's interest in the patient and to assist him to develop awareness regarding behavior, thereby re-establishing contact with reality
Elicit patient's feelings regarding the problem behavior.	to bring feelings into awareness so that coping mechanisms can be developed
Identify the precipitating cause of aggressive behavior with the patient.	to determine the purpose of the patient's behavior so that the nurse can choose the best method of intervention
Devise and explore alternative behavioral responses.	to assist the patient to develop socially acceptable patterns of behaving
Provide distraction and channel aggressive behavior through mildly competitive games like cards, checkers, chess; constructive tasks; and challenging activities at which the patient is known to be proficient.	to provide socially acceptable outlets for the expression of aggressive behavior, to foster self-esteem and to promote feelings of accomplishment and independence
Apply external controls (as a last resort) such as direct verbal commands ("Stop yelling!"); impose consequences for unmet expectations ("If you don't stop banging the table, you'll have to go back to your room"); and exert direct physical control by laying on hands using medicinal or mechanical restraints.	to provide protection and control for the patient until such time as he is able to exert self-control

manipulative behavior

Manipulative behavior is control behavior. Through manipulative behavior, an individual uses others to meet his own needs or to achieve his goals. Manipulative behavior is used to disguise the individual's underlying feelings of inadequacy, inferiority and unworthiness. Its use by the individual is an attempt to protect himself against failure or frustration and to gain power over another. This maladaptive behavior has a depersonalizing effect on others and tends to evoke strong, negative feelings on the part of the respondent. These negative feelings are conveyed through dislike, disbelief, rejection, retaliation or punishment. Such responses tend to reinforce the individual's dependency, increase his anxiety and foster continued use of and reliance on manipulative behavior as a mode of adaptation.

One of the frequently overlooked effects of the patient's manipulative behavior is the engendering of negativism and parallel manipulative behavior by the staff. Often the staff reacts to the manipulative, angry patient, with his incessant demands, unrealistic expectations of the staff, endless complaints against the institution and the care given by assuming that the patient's behavior and verbal expressions are a direct, personal affront. Consequently, the staff singles out the manipulative patient as "a troublemaker," "a chronic complainer," "an inappropriate admission" and other derogatory terms that result in subconscious sabotage of treatment interventions and disinterest in patient-care outcomes. The self and subsequent understanding of the self, as discussed in Chapter Three, is of fundamental importance when approaching the manipulative patient. The approach best suited for creating a therapeutic environment for individuals with manipulative behavior is one that is firm, kind, consistent, matter-of-fact and realistic. It is vitally important to the therapeutic process and the successful treatment of the manipulative patient that a consistent approach be rendered on a twenty-four-hour basis. This necessitates that the nurse must be clear, concise and complete in her report to others regarding modifications of the patient's behavior, additions to or deletions from the original treatment approach and must share the contributions made by other disciplines in the implementation and evaluation of the contract. The significant attitudes necessary for the implementation of this approach are integrity, openmindedness, personal worth and nonpunitiveness.

Specific interventions the nurse can use to deal effectively with manipulative behavior are listed in Table 17-4.

TABLE 17-4
MANIPULATIVE BEHAVIOR—INTERVENTION AND RATIONALE

Intervention	Rationale
Observe the particular way the patient's manipulative behavior is manifest.	to provide information needed for appropriate intervention
Observe the reactions of self and others to the manipulative behavior.	to prevent other patients, the nurses or other team members from becoming trapped by the manipulative behavior

TABLE 17-4 (continued)

Intervention	Rationale
Identify feelings engendered within the nurse by the manipulative behavior.	to create awareness and self-understanding so that appropriate, therapeutic interruption of the manipulative cycle can be effected
Recognize instances in which the patient is using manipulative behavior.	to avoid being used as a tool by the patient and to promote the patient's awareness of his behavior
Refrain from responding or being "taken in" by manipulative behavior such as teasing, personal remarks designed to flatter or embarrass and vulgar language or risque jokes.	to prevent the continuation of the manipulative pattern and to prevent reinforcement of the patient's negative view of self
Identify limits for the patient which the staff is willing to accept.	to formulate positive expectations and prevent "unconscious sabotage" of the therapeutic plan by the patient or the staff
Explain to the patient first, positive expectations, and second, the extent of the limits.	to overcome the pattern of failure and decrease frustration
Recognize the patient's repeated attempts at testing limits.	to develop the nurse's awareness, promote her understanding and to interrupt the patient's manipulative pattern
Implement consistency and elicit the cooperation of all team members.	to interrupt the manipulative behavior pattern, reduce anxiety and increase the patient's potential for cooperating with the therapeutic regime
Provide continuity of approach, expectations and limits on a twenty-four-hour basis.	to increase the patient's awareness and need for consistent controls on his own behavior and to assist the patient to learn to delay immediate need gratification
Listen and respond openly, directly and honestly without expressing anger, disappointment or disgust.	to build the individual's healthy concept of self and what is acceptable, social behavior
Assist the patient to learn to use the problem solving approach in his relationship with others.	to help the patient to learn self-control and to accept the concept of cooperation, collaboration and compromise

self-destructive behavior

Self-destructive behavior is revengeful, angry self-punishment. Self-destructive behavior is carried out by those individuals who believe they have failed to live up to the ideals and expectations they have set up for themselves or believe others require of them. They experience this pseudofailure in terms of radically lowered self-esteem and pervasive, personal inadequacy. They express their feelings in terms of uncertainty, helplessness, hopelessness and vitriolic self-criticism. Underlying self-desctructive behavior are tremendous feelings of anger, disappointment, resentment and hostility. Through the self-destructive behavior, the individual attempts to strike out against and eradicate that part of the self that is so unpleasant, unrewarding, impotent and ineffective. The self-destructive individual is so preoccupied with retaliation against the self and others that he is unable to formulate effective, satisfying interpersonal ties or glean satisfaction from any achievements. Self-destructive acts include such behaviors as continuous scratching or picking at self; a seeming ignorance or unawareness of environmental hazards; repeated accidents, illness, and injuries; high alcohol or drug consumption and suicidal thoughts or attempts. This type of behavior creates within the observer a feeling of dislike, disgust, repulsion and rejection. This response on the part of staff occurs because the physical sight of self-inflicted injury is in itself distressing, and because of the possible feelings of personal threat such acts provoke.

The twentieth century will be noted for the prevalence of depression. It permeates every segment of civilized society, irrespective of class, race or culture. Nursing personnel within institutions, hospitals and other patient care facilities are constantly confronted with the problem of intervening, managing and delivering interventive techniques for patients manifesting self-destructive behaviors. In Chapter Fourteen we dealt with depression, its symptomology and dynamics. The reader will find that reviewing this chapter will be informative and helpful in understanding the self-destructive patient.

The creation of a therapeutic atmosphere must include an approach which is gentle, warm and accepting. The attitudes necessary to implement this approach are hopefulness, personal worth and involvement.

Specific interventions the nurse can use to interrupt self-destructive behavior are listed in Table 17-5.

TABLE 17-5
SELF-DESTRUCTIVE BEHAVIOR—INTERVENTION AND RATIONALE

Intervention	Rationale
Pay close attention to family and personal history.	to make assessment of suicide potential
Assess suicide potential.	to alert the health team and determine the immediate goal for intervention
Listen carefully to delusional or hallucinatory content.	to pick up cues regarding increases in the level and intensity of anxiety or fear
Listen to verbal communication for possible threats, plans or decisions about death or dying.	to demonstrate interest and concern and to gather data for immediate crisis intervention
Observe patient behavior closely for changes in mood, appetite, drives, levels of energy or concentration.	to provide data with which to evaluate suicide potential and plan necessary intervention

TABLE 17-5 (continued)

Intervention	Rationale
Make rounds at frequent irregular intervals, particularly during the night, toward early morning at change of shift or during "busy times" for unit personnel.	to prevent, interfere with or interrupt any destructive behavior
Assign patient to a room close to the nurse's station.	to increase nurse's accessibility to the patient and to increase opportunities for observation
Maintain distance and interaction between patients exhibiting similar behaviors.	to prevent these patients from reinforcing each other's self-destructive behavior
Decrease environmental hazards such as sharp instruments, cleaning supplies, belts, cords, electrical equipment or drugs.	to provide safety and protection for the patient and to provide reassurance that someone cares and that the staff will not permit him to be self-destructive
Plan for and assign the patient to menial but useful tasks—scrubbing sinks in the bathroom, scouring ashtrays, cleaning water fountains, emptying trash cans.	to relieve guilt, satisfy the need for "punishment" and to provide opportunity for increase in self-esteem through accomplishment of necessary and worthwhile activity
Limit possibilities of body contact when engaging in recreational, occupational or work activities.	to prevent the displacement of anger or hostility onto others in the immediate environment, to decrease the potential for impulsive acting out and to prevent bodily injury to others
Redirect expressions of anger or hostility into acceptable channels; for example, bowling, typing, playing the piano, tearing strips of cloth to be used in weaving or as fillers for stuffed toys or pillows.	to prevent the negative feelings from being directed towards self or objects and to encourage and reinforce the use of alternatives to destructive behavior
Insure that the patient is not left alone.	to decrease the patient's feelings that no one cares, to minimize the opportunities for destructive behavior and to provide an opportunity for close observation without hovering
Seek out the patient at frequent intervals and then gradually introduce him to others.	to develop closeness between the patient and the nurse, to demonstrate to the patient the nurse's respect for his importance as a person and to supply opportunities for the development of potentially meaningful interpersonal relationships without overwhelming him
Be sincere and honest with the patient: "We will not permit you to harm yourself," or, "Yes, we are interested in where you are and what you are doing."	to demonstrate respect, acceptance and a sincere appreciation for his personal worth
Inaugurate a "busy" schedule.	to keep the patient occupied and to prevent preoccupation with self-destructive thoughts or behavior

TABLE 17-5 (continued)

Intervention	Rationale
Alert all personnel to the patient's self-destructive behavior.	to minimize hazards, to promote safety and to provide continuity of concerned care
Implement definite limits or restrictions on mobility or whereabouts; for example, accompany the patient to all off-ward activity, assign one member of the staff to be responsible for close unobtrusive observation or supervise the patient's use of potentially hazardous equipment.	to decrease the patient's potential accessibility to environmental hazards
Permit the patient to verbalize suicidal threats, do not ignore them; do not argue with the patient about them; and take his statements seriously.	to establish trust, to recognize the importance of the intent and to determine the time when protective action is most needed
Encourage the patient to make simple decisions according to his capabilities such as what to wear or eat, whether to watch T.V. or play cards.	to foster a sense of accomplishment and self-control, and to exercise independent functioning
Make all other decisions for the patient.	to eliminate overwhelming anxiety and thereby reduce the patient's need to engage in self-destructive behavior as the only avenue of escape
Remain calm, unimpressed but not indifferent to self-destructive activity.	to provide a feeling of security, to minimize the patient's fear and guilt and to reduce the possibility of successful completion of the suicidal act
Convey warmth and interest in the patient but not in the suicidal act or threat; for example: "You've hurt yourself, it must be painful, let me help you."	to demonstrate acceptance of the person, to display a nonjudgmental attitude toward the person and to convey concern and understanding
Avoid angry, critical comments which might be interpreted by the patient as a dare, threat or "calling his bluff" such as, "Don't you know that dose wouldn't have killed you" and "You severed a vein, not an artery."	to prevent reinforcement of guilt and further decrease in self-esteem
Interrupt self-destructive acts by placing a protective arm about the patient, suggesting that the patient talk the situation over, diverting attention from the suicidal act toward something else, making an appeal to reason or persuading the patient to postpone his suicidal action.	to prevent death, to allow time for interpersonal techniques to be employed and to determine underlying causative factors for the particular self-destructive behavior
Pay attention to physical needs by encouraging adequate nutritional intake, observing response to drug therapy, closely observing patient's ingestion of medication, promoting adequate rest and sleep and preventing fatigue.	to promote and maintain physiological functioning

hyperactive behavior

Hyperactive behavior is exaggerated behavior. It is an irrational, excessive response to stimuli. The hyperactive individual reacts impulsively and forcefully to people, places and things. Hyperactivity is an attempt on the part of the individual to exercise control and dominance over the environment. Furthermore, this individual is unable to concentrate. Symptomatically, this means that the patient makes loose associations or displays a short attention span. The inability to concentrate precludes effective listening and communication. In addition, his pattern of speech is often fragmented and nonsequential which indicates the stream of stimuli that he is evidently internalizing and to which he is outwardly responding. Hyperactivity is overcompensatory behavior used to mask the individual's feelings of inferiority, inadequacy, inability to perform and to relate meaningfully to others. The hyperactive individual is angry, fearful and in a constant state of threat. This hyperactivity is demonstrated through accelerated psychomotor activity, increase in physical prowess and hyperventilation. The hyperactive individual is easily irritated and excited and given to wide mood swings, capriciousness, distractability and destructiveness.

A quiet, firm, kind, persuasive approach is most effective in dealing with hyperactive behavior. The attitudes most needed by the nurse to implement the approach are advocacy, openmindedness, personal worth, and calm, temperate firmness.

Specific interventions the nurse can employ to deal with hyperactive behavior are listed in Table 17-6.

TABLE 17-6
HYPERACTIVE BEHAVIOR—INTERVENTION AND RATIONALE

Intervention	Rationale
Provide a subdued environment, remove unnecessary furniture, take pictures off walls, tone down bright, harsh colors and eliminate excess noise.	to reduce sensory input to decrease hyperactivity
Assign patient to private room.	to provide him with a quiet area to reduce environmental and interpersonal stimulation
Reduce the number of contacts the patient has with people, assign the same staff members to him, discourage visitations from other patients, relatives and personnel and limit the patient's participation with groups.	to decrease irritability, to decrease impulsive interaction, to prevent attempts at dominating others, to protect the patient from retaliation from others and to promote physical distance which helps lessen misidentification of "approach" behavior as "attack" behavior
Monitor food intake.	to maintain nutritional needs and to plan and provide necessary adjustments in dietary intake
Provide a high caloric, high vitamin diet with supplemental feedings.	to combat exhaustion and weight loss due to high energy output

TABLE 17-6 (continued)

Intervention	Rationale
Provide finger foods such as sandwiches, cookies, fruit, milk shakes.	to provide foods which can be eaten as the patient moves about because he is "too busy" to sit down and eat
Increase fluid intake.	to prevent dehydration and constipation and to assist in elimination of medication to prevent toxicity
Initiate weight chart.	to monitor possible weight loss
Supervise personal hygiene: assist with collection of necessary toilet articles, adjust temperature of shower or bath water; assist and instruct patient with bathing, oral hygiene, shaving, dressing; observe condition of skin and general state of the body for injury or misuse; and control the patient's use of toiletries, cosmetics and jewelry.	to maintain physical well-being, to combat disorganization and distractibility, to provide for safety needed because of the patient's poor judgment, to insure cleanliness, neatness and appropriateness, to prevent patient from being an object of ridicule and to promote positive self-image
Encourage the patient to wear his own clothes.	to maintain identity and contact with reality
Maintain patient's wardrobe—keep clothing in good repair, advise and provide changes of attire according to season, activity and time of day, remove from pockets accumulated junk or items which belong to others.	to encourage appropriateness of appearance and to maintain identity and to set realistic limits
Monitor physiological functioning: observe for signs and symptoms of physical distress, encourage patient to verbalize discomforts, investigate record and report somatic complaints.	to maintain a state of physiological homeostasis and guard against illness and to intervene and prevent the development of any pathophysiological condition
Exercise vigilance in administration of medication: if the patient refuses the medication, don't argue, distract his attention while offering the medication; if the patient seeks to postpone taking medication, go on to the next patient in line and then return using positive suggestions, "It's now time to take your medication"; if patient is hoarding, closely observe for swallowing, increase fluids, inspect his mouth, change to liquid or parenteral administration.	to maintain effective therapeutic drug regime or to prevent possible misuse of drugs by the patient or others
Promote rest and sleep by observing usual sleep patterns; reducing stimuli prior to bed time; using somatic comfort measures like hot tubs, warm milk, back rubs; administering prescribed medication; and prescribing and planning for daily rest period.	to prevent fatigue, exhaustion and circulatory collapse

TABLE 17-6 (continued)

Intervention	Rationale
Provide a regular supervised, noncompetitive, solitary or small group activity such as swimming, gymnastics, walking, running, housekeeping, raking grass, finger painting or writing.	to direct excessive amount of energy into appropriate channels, to increase sedentary activity to prevent fatigue and to lessen hyperactive behavior and allow for expression of angry feelings
Select projects or activities which can be completed in a short time.	to provide opportunities for the patient to experience success, to counteract feelings of inferiority and inadequacy and to assist the patient to develop self-control
Listen quietly and attentively to the patient.	to act as a sounding board for his excitement
Attempt to interrupt flow of conversation.	to refocus on "real" concerns
Schedule short, frequent interaction sessions.	to make maximum use of the patient's short attention span
Give short, simple, direct explanations for procedures and activities.	to maintain focus on reality
Observe for changes in mood and behavior such as increasing irritability and increased physical or verbal activity.	to assess the need for specific intervention and to prevent hyperactive crisis
Define firm, consistent limits for the patient.	to establish external control and to aid in the prevention of hyperactive crisis
Guard against becoming maneuvered by the patient's excitement, impetuosity, grandiosity and hyperactivity.	to prevent loss of personal control and therapeutic effectiveness

compulsive behavior

Compulsive behavior is stereotyped behavior. It is peculiar, repetitive behavior. The individual is usually intellectually cognizant that his behavior is exaggerated, impulsive, inappropriate and undesirable. Nevertheless, he is unable to stop and feels compelled to carry out the ritualistic, repetitive act. With this type of behavior the individual disguises his overwhelming anxiety. Each repetitive act is significant for the individual and its form of expression is directly related to the particular problem producing the anxiety. The majority of ritualistic acts are in effect "make-up" behaviors. The individual is attempting to atone for past or present guilt feelings either by restitution or undoing. The nurse's approach should include kind, patient acceptance and understanding. The attitudes the nurse needs to implement in this approach are integrity, personal worth, openmindedness and involvement.

Specific interventions the nurse can employ to deal with compulsive behavior are listed in Table 17-7.

TABLE 17-7
COMPULSIVE BEHAVIOR—INTERVENTION AND RATIONALE

Intervention	Rationale
Modify environment, schedules and routines.	to convey acceptance, to permit the patient time to carry out his ritualistic behavior without interruption and to reduce his anxiety
Plan, discuss and implement with the patient an individualized schedule of daily activities.	to accomodate his need for repetitive acts and to demonstrate support for the patient
Expect patient to adhere to planned schedule which includes time for ritualistic behavior as well as consistent limits on the behavior.	to convey acceptance and understanding by not subjecting the individual to ridicule or criticism and to meet needs through alternative means
Anticipate needs by offering self through frequent, planned contact; listening to and encouraging verbalization; administering medication *on time*; and giving information, instructions, or items for daily living, before he has to ask.	to increase feelings of security, reduce anxiety and demonstrate personal worth and integrity
Plan and participate in diversional activity with the patient.	to prevent preoccupation with self and to substitute more appropriate means for reducing anxiety
Choose recreational and occupational therapy according to old interests and successful accomplishments.	to insure success and positive feedback which increase his self-image
Introduce patient to small group activity.	to release tension and provide new interests and to meet the needs for affection, recognition and belonging
Seek out and spend time with the patient.	provide the patient with therapeutic support which allays feelings of guilt and anxiety
Listen patiently and attentively to verbalization of feelings.	to convey acceptance and interest
Focus communication on problem areas.	to assist the patient with identification and to develop awareness of anxiety and conflict
Explore current conflict in relationship to ritualistic behavior.	to facilitate comparison and to encourage decision making
Support decisions made and assist the patient to implement new behaviors.	to interrupt the use of ritualistic behavior, to promote psychological comfort and to provide necessary reassurance to lessen anxiety
Observe for signs of mounting anxiety and intervene before the patient resorts to ritualistic behaviors.	to prevent the need for the behavior pattern and to assist the patient to learn to deal with anxiety

addictive behavior

Addictive behavior is flight from pain and a search for pleasure. It is the manifestation of altered physiological and psychological processes which results in dependency on substances that permit the individual to escape, avoid, distort, obliterate or escalate his thoughts, feelings and/or actions. Substances used to produce major physiological and psychological alterations include alcohol, hallucinogenic agents, narcotics, sedatives, stimulants and volatile chemicals. The type of substance taken, its availability, and motivating factors differ with each abuser.

Addictive behavior is one of the most prevalent, disruptive phenomena invading all strata of society. There are many forms of addiction from the most common and socially acceptable addiction to caffeine as illustrated by the "universal coffee break" to the more bizarre, socially unacceptable and often destructive misuse and abuse of hallucinogenic agents. The results are unmistakable whether one is young or old, rich or poor, male or female. Prolonged abuse eventuates in both the physical and mental deterioration of the individual; causes serious disruption and often produces seemingly irreconcilable conflicts within family units and directly or indirectly negatively affects society at large.

Addictive behavior is used by the individual as a means of changing his present reality. It is used as a prop for hope and happiness. It involves the seeking after a state of well-being in which all problems, needs, wants and desires disappear, are magically resolved or are relegated to a position of secondary importance. As a means to an end, addictive behavior is a substitute for problem-solving and confrontation with reality. The individual uses his addiction much like the circus clown uses his "paint pots," that is, to mask his real self from the real world. The mask enables the abuser to be or not to be! It allows him to present to the world an outward show of bravado or confidence that he does not feel or that does not exist. It permits him to display outgoing or assertive behavior which covers his inner timidity or fearfulness. It enables him to deny, rationalize and project his ideas or actions in an effort to conceal and protect himself from assuming responsibility for self and involvement with others. It lets him manifest exaggerated feeling states to relieve the discomfort of perceived boredom, routine or loneliness. The drug abuser is firmly convinced that the drug route is the only avenue open to him in his fight for survival.

Reluctance, opposition, open conflict and defiance of all authority are predominant behavioral characteristics of the drug abuser. This individual plays games, is a master in the art of manipulation and uses others to achieve his own ends. The addicted individual is a person whose tolerance for stress is minimal, whose ego strengths are few and whose ability to cope is almost non-existent. The predominantly aggressive tactics used by the drug abuser, namely, subtle inuendos; abusive, insulting language; loud, demanding, threatening verbalizations; or intimidating gestures are essentially distancing manuevers which segregate him from society and prevent the development of close, warm, human ties.

A firm, consistent, matter-of-fact and realistic approach is essential for individuals who manifest addictive behavior. The significant attitudes which must be cultivated by the nurse in implementing this approach are integrity, personal worth, open-mindedness and non-punitiveness. Specific interventions the nurse might consider to deal with the problem of addictive behavior are included in the following charts. The interventions are divided according to the three essential phases of the treatment process: detoxification, rehabilitation, and follow-up. See Table 17-8.

TABLE 17-8
NURSING INTERVENTION IN ADDICTIVE BEHAVIOR
DETOXIFICATION

Intervention	Rationale
Assign the same staff on a prolonged basis and initiate a therapeutic nurse-patient relationship	to provide consistency, reduce fear and allow for development of trust
Remain with patient and exercise close observation	to monitor changes in patient status; to collect data for reassessing and up-dating of the care plan; to offer reassurance; to provide additional emotional support and, limit access to abused drug
Take vital signs frequently and accurately	to establish a data base and to prevent complications
Monitor intake and output	to maintain hydration and to observe for retention
Note response to questions and directions	to determine alterations in levels of consciousness and to identify the presence of psychopathological symptomatology
Note changes in behavior	to intiate preventive measures thereby safeguarding the patient from experiencing the acute discomfort frequently associated with withdrawal
Check and relay laboratory findings to physician	to keep physician informed of serum electrolyte imbalance
Document and report changes in patient status immediately	to prevent crisis
Check personal belongings of patient	to ensure that patient or others have not secreted a supply of abused drug
Restrict or limit visitors	to prevent or reduce potential hazard of obtaining abused drugs from outside sources

REHABILITATION

Intervention	Rationale
Continue therapeutic relationship initiated during detoxification	to continue identification of problems, needs and concerns; to set realistic

TABLE 17-8 (continued)

Intervention	Rationale
	goals and explore alternatives to addictive patterns of behavior
Involve the patient in developing and adjusting an on-going plan of care	to foster the patient's sense of responsibility and accountability in the management of his own treatment; to acknowledge the patient's right to have input into his own care
Structure activities of daily living	to provide consistency and to limit the amount of unplanned "free" time
Set and maintain limits	to provide consistency, maintain structure and minimize manipulative behavior
Provide a variety of group experiences relating to: work opportunities; drug abuse education; social interaction; gripes and unmet needs; discharge planning and community placement	to increase interpersonal contact; to share, compare and verify interpersonal experiences; to develop group communication skills and socialization; to assist the patient to begin movement toward independent functioning; to provide another avenue for continued growth and responsibility; and, to support and reinforce abstinence behavior
Insist on active participation in total treatment plan	to motivate the patient; to present reality; to reduce potential manipulative behavior; and, assess commitment to treatment process
Include family members, relatives or friends in the treatment plan	to provide support to patient and family; to enlist cooperation of significant others
Implement a mechanism for checking patient's whereabouts at all times	to maintain supervision and observational processes and to provide additional data for evaluating the effectiveness of care

FOLLOW-UP

Intervention	Rationale
Maintain therapeutic relationship with original staff	to provide continuity of care
Plan with patient a detailed schedule for: out-patient clinic visits; individual counseling; group sessions; home visits; family counseling	to provide structure, consistency and support in assisting the patient and his family to meet the demands of adjustment outside the hospital environment; to monitor physical change; to foster and sustain continuous movement toward independent functioning and to reduce possibility of potential relapse

suspicious behavior

Suspicious behavior is forceful, aggressive, confrontation toward others. Such behavior is manifested through a consistent, persistent tendency to doubt and to mistrust the sincerity, motivation, reliability or honesty of others. In his relationship with others, the suspicious individual makes no allowance for human error. Suspicious behavior is compensatory behavior used to disguise, project or deny feelings of insecurity, interpersonal inadequacy and distortions of personal identity. Often the psychotically suspicious patient manifests his internal response to hallucinatory experiences through his observable behavior. These hallucinatory experiences may be auditory, visual, gustatory, tactile or olfactory. Each of the experiences lends itself to the creation of additional suspicion and mistrust of other people, his environment and the objects within his immediate or remote surroundings. This heightened suspiciousness intensifies the patient's already overwhelming feelings of insecurity. As a result the suspicious individual feels isolated, lonely, fearful and anxious. Examples of suspicious behavior include spreading of dissatisfaction; subtle sabotage; dissemination of evil tidings or pessimistic warnings; portrayal of pretentious, dramatic self-sacrifice; spreading harmful tales about others or inciting violence. For patients who display suspicious behavior a kind, helpful, nonthreatening and somewhat detached approach by the nurse, along with attitudes of personal worth, hopefulness and integrity produce the needed therapeutic environment.

Specific interventions the nurse can use to deal with suspicious behavior are listed in Table 17-9.

TABLE 17-9
SUSPICIOUS BEHAVIOR—INTERVENTION AND RATIONALE

Intervention	Rationale
Be frank, open and honest.	to counteract the patient's mistrust
Demonstrate dependability through keeping promises, being on time for appointments and alerting the patient well in advance of schedule changes.	to establish trust and integrity
Clarify and restate role; repeat with patience and understanding.	to prevent misinterpretations, to decrease fear of involvement, to establish trust and, to define the helping relationship
Listen for expressions of fear, anxiety and mistrust in communications.	to identify and help the patient recognize problems
Reflect and explore feelings.	to identify and clarify the relationship between feeling and behavior
Discuss, implement and evaluate with the patient alternatives for suspicious behavior.	to produce behavioral change and to demonstrate to the patient a satisfactory method of adaptation through the use of problem solving

TABLE 17-9 (continued)

Intervention	Rationale
Minimize contact with staff.	to protect the patient from feeling threatened by too much interpersonal contact
Eliminate unnecessary physical contact—do not touch the patient.	to avoid misinterpretation of action as an attack on the patient
Assign to solitary, noncompetitive activity such as messenger or escort service, picture puzzles, weaving, drawing, photography and typing.	to minimize feelings of insecurity or inferiority
Allow patient the freedom to select activities within the scope of available choices.	to decrease mistrust and to foster a potential sense of accomplishment
Reward completion of meaningful tasks with merited praise.	to increase self-esteem and to promote a more realistic view of self
Be alert and observe for potential problem areas in eating, sleeping and the taking of medications.	to plan intervention before the problem becomes unmanageable

suggested readings

Almeida, Elza M., and Chapman A. H. *The Interpersonal Basis of Psychiatric Nursing*. G. P. Putman's Sons: New York, 1972.

Anders, Robert L. "When a Patient Becomes Violent." *American Journal of Nursing*, Vol. 77 No. 7 (July, 1977), 1144-48.

Briggs, Paulette Fitzgerald. "Specializing in Psychiatry: Therapeutic or Custodial?" *Nursing Outlook*, Vol. 22 No. 10 (October, 1974), 632-635.

Cavers, Annie, and Williams, Robert. "The Budget Plan (Behavior Modification of Long-Term Patients)." *Perspectives in Psychiatric Care*, Vol. 9 No. 1 (January, 1971), 13-16.

_____. "Dealing With Rage." *Nursing '75*, Vol. 5 No. 10 (October, 1975), 25-29.

Fernandez, Theresa M. "How to Deal With Overt Aggression." *American Journal of Nursing*, Vol. 59 No. 5 (May, 1959), 658-660.

Glasser, William. *Reality Therapy*. Harper & Row: New York, 1975.

Goldstein, Sheila. "Impulse Control." *Journal of Psychiatric Nursing and Mental Health Services*, Vol. 14 No. 7 (July, 1976), 36-40.

Jurgensen, Kathleen. "Limit Setting for Hospitalized Adolescent Psychiatric Patients." *Perspectives in Psychiatric Care*, Vol. 9 No. 4 (1971), 173-182.

Kolb, Lawrence C. *Noyes' Modern Clinical Psychiatry*. 7th ed. W. B. Saunders Co.: Philadelphia, 1968.

Lamb, Dorothy E. "Nurse–Geriatric Patients Relationships in a Stress Situation."

Phases in Human Development: Relevance in Nursing. American Nurses Association: New York, 1962, 30-38.

LeBow, Michael D. *Behavior Modification.* Prentice Hall Inc.: Englewood Cliffs, New Jersey, 1973.

Loomis, Maxine E. "Nursing Management of Acting Out Behavior." *Perspectives in Psychiatric Care*, Vol. 8 No. 4 (1970), 168-173.

Nelson, Priscilla. "Involvement with Betty: An Experience in Reality Therapy." *American Journal of Nursing*, Vol. 74 No. 8 (August, 1974), 1440-1441.

Royalty, Debbie Casey. " 'Try to Help Her Keep Her Clothes On.' That Was the Staff's Only Goal." *Nursing '76*, Vol. 6 No. 4 (April, 1976), 38-40.

Scheideman, Jean. "Remotivation: Involvement Without Labels." *Journal of Psychiatric Nursing and Mental Health Services*, Vol. 14 No. 7 (July, 1976), 41-42.

Schwartz, Morris S., and Shockley, Emmy Lanning. *The Nurse and The Mental Patient.* Russell Sage Foundation: New York, 1956.

Swanson, Ardis. "The Self-Fulfilling Prophesy in Schizophrenia." *Exploring Progress in Psychiatric Nursing Practice*. American Nurses Association: New York, 1965, 26-32.

chapter 18

nursing intervention for patients experiencing procedure-oriented activity

learning objectives

On completion of this chapter the reader should be able to:

1 Define *procedure-oriented activity*.

2 Recognize and understand the nurse's role in carrying out procedure-oriented activity.

3 Understand the purpose and expected therapeutic results of chemotherapy, activity therapy and electro-convulsive therapy.

4 Identify potential or existing nursing care problems for the patient receiving these therapies.

5 Select specific interventions for prevention or resolution of the identified problem.

6 Explain the rationale upon which the interventions are based.

In this chapter we address ourselves to three frequently used procedure-oriented activities—chemotherapy, activity therapy and electro-convulsive therapy (ECT), any or all of which may be included as part of a patient's total treatment program. We define a *procedure-oriented activity* as an adjunctive treatment modality in which physical manipulation of the patient's internal and external environment produces both a physical response as well as a social and psychological change in the patient's perceptions of self and others. Although these procedure-oriented activities commonly take place within the hospital setting, they may also be carried out in such treatment settings as a physician's office, a mental health clinic or in an outpatient department. To achieve therapeutic effectiveness these procedure-oriented activities need the patient's full cooperation and participation; therefore, the primary nursing care goal is *to secure, promote and maintain the patient's collaborative assistance.*

psychotropic chemotherapy

Psychotropic chemotherapy is an adjunctive treatment which produces a relief of symptoms, thereby enabling the patient to make maximum use of the total treatment regime. Specifically, it is used to bring about changes in an individual's disrupted thinking, distorted feelings and disturbed behavior. Those chemical agents that fall within this classification are the major and minor tranquilizers, and antidepressants and the antihallucinogenic agents. These psychotropic agents are directly responsible for alleviating anxiety, decreasing psychomotor activity, increasing perception, decreasing depression and interrupting psychotic symptomology. These changes foster an attitude conducive to psychotherapeutic intervention in the form of individual or group psychotherapy.

This section is intended to increase the knowledge and skill of the nurse in the administration and monitoring of drugs and in assessing the patient's response behavior, that is, determining the therapeutic effectiveness of the drug. For information regarding specific drugs, the reader is referred to current pharmacology textbooks, handbooks, pharmaceutical literature and journal articles.

The nurse should be aware that drug therapy is not to be considered a panacea for the patient's problems. Neither should it be a replacement for good clinical practice or a routine procedure carried on without sound clinical judgment. Therefore, the nurse's approach to the patient undergoing chemotherapy should be one that is knowledgeable, firm, confident and actively observant. To achieve this approach the nurse must cultivate the attitudes of involvement, hopefulness, openmindedness and advocacy.

Specific interventions designed to assist patients undergoing chemotherapy are listed in Table 18-1.

TABLE 18-1
PSYCHOTROPIC CHEMOTHERAPY—INTERVENTION AND RATIONALE

Intervention	Rationale
Be *aware* of the specific drugs prescribed for the patient.	to make accurate assessment of the effectiveness of chemotherapy
Be *familiar* with the purpose for which the specific drug is prescribed.	to give meaning and purpose for the interpreations of the clinical observation
Be *alert* to the action, desired effects, usual dosage, side effects, contradiction, precautions and nursing implications related to the prescribed drug.	to exercise vigilance on behalf of the patient in order to protect him and to maintain his physical comfort and well-being

TABLE 18-1 (continued)

Intervention	Rationale
Instruct the patient and his family members about the patient's drug therapy program including the name of the drug, usual side effects, danger signals and comfort measures.	to secure the patient's and the family's cooperation through education to decrease anxiety for all
Elicit and explore with the patient his thoughts and feelings regarding taking the prescribed medications.	to identify his value system, to determine his level of understanding, to provide support and to alleviate fear and anxiety
Answer the patient's drug-related questions openly and honestly.	to establish trust, to provide the patient with correct information and to clarify misinterpretations
Administer the prescribed medication to the right patient, in the right dose at the right time and use the right route of administration.	to protect the patient's right to quality treatment and care
Administer antidepressants to later than 5:00 p.m.	to prevent insomnia
Plan to observe the patient and evaluate the clinical effectiveness of the patient's drug program.	to determine the patient's response to drug therapy and to provide a data base for making recommendations for change in the nursing care and treatment plan
Encourage the patient to promptly report untoward reactions.	to provide protection and implement appropriate nursing intervention

stumbling blocks and stepping stones

There is an abundance of reference material on psychotropic drugs and chemotherapy readily available to the nurse. This material supplies information on effects, side effects, untoward reactions and contradications. But information related to necessary precautions and specific nursing interventions is limited. Therefore, we identify some of the more common problems, or stumbling blocks, encountered and provide some suggestions, or stepping stones for effective intervention. These are as follows listed in Table 18-2.

TABLE 18-2
COMMON STUMBLING BLOCKS AND STEPPING STONES
ASSOCIATED WITH CHEMOTHERAPY

STUMBLING BLOCKS	STEPPING STONES
"What if—	Try this—
1) the patient complains of dizziness?	Change the patient's position slowly.
	Lower the patient's head down between his knees.
	Instruct patient to remain in a recumbent position one-half to one hour after parenteral administration.

TABLE 18-2 (continued)

STUMBLING BLOCKS	STEPPING STONES
"What if—	*Try this—*
	Check and record blood pressure.
	Have the patient sit down periodically.
	Instruct the patient to walk close to the walls in corridors.
	Note frequency and duration of the complaint.
2) the patient complains of a dry mouth?	Have the patient take frequent *small*, sips of water.
	Suggest sucking ice chips or hard *sour* candies.
	Suggest chewing gum.
	Have the patient rinse his mouth frequently.
	Lubricate the patient's lips.
3) the patient complains of blurred vision?	Provide adequate lighting.
	Provide large print books and newspapers.
	Have the patient read with a light over his right shoulder.
	Recommend an opthalmological consultation and periodic eye examination.
4) the patient has slurred speech?	Listen carefully and patiently.
	Encourage the patient to speak slowly.
	Ask him to repeat when necessary.
5) the patient has an unsteady gait?	Instruct the patient to walk slowly.
	Encourage him to wear sturdy, supportive shoes.
	Show him how to use his arms for balance and support.
	Have him use railings and walls for support.
	Provide a cane or walker if necessary.
	Remind and encourage him to walk erectly.
	Assist and supervise ambulation.
6) the patient gains weight?	Keep a weight record.
	Reduce his caloric intake.
	Discourage and restrict his eating "junk foods."
	Discourage and restrict his eating between meals.
7) the patient complains of drowsiness?	Discourage staying in bed all day.
	Plan schedules so that major activities occur immediately after drug administration.

TABLE 18-2 (continued)

STUMBLING BLOCKS	STEPPING STONES
"What if—	*Try this—*
	Include time for rest periods in the patient's schedule.
8) the patient has edema?	Check intake and output.
	Restrict fluid intake.
	Instruct the patient to elevate his legs periodically.
9) the patient experiences photosensitivity?	Provide patient with protective clothing to cover exposed skin areas.
	Encourage him to wear a wide-brimmed hat outdoors.
	Advise him to keep out of direct rays of sun.
	Apply *sun screening* lotion to his exposed areas.
	Plan for and encourage indoor activities.
10) the patient complains of sore throat, runny nose or cold?	Check vital signs.
	Observe and report the condition of his throat.
	Report symptoms to physician.
	Initiate laboratory request to check for agranulocytosis.
11) the patient experiences drooling, twitching of face muscles, swelling and protrusion of tongue?	Alert physician immediately.
	Withhold drug.
	Observe patient closely while waiting for physician's intervention.
	Force fluids.
	Maintain patent airway.
	Administer oxygen.
12) the patient experiences anorexia, nausea or other gastro-intestinal symptoms?	Restrict food high in fats and carbohydrates.
	Give medication with skim milk.
	Plan for small, frequent feedings.
	Observe closely for jaundice.
13) the patient complains of feeling cold?	Provide proper clothing.
	Check temperature periodically.
	Regulate temperature of bath water.
	Advise patient to be cautious in handling hot coffee, tea, water; to avoid direct contact with radiators, hot water bottles or heating pads.
14) the patient complains of constipation?	Increase roughage, bulk and fluid intake.
	Check frequency and consistency of stool.

TABLE 18-2 (continued)

STUMBLING BLOCKS	STEPPING STONES
"What if—	*Try this—*
	Encourage the patient to increase physical exercise.
15) the patient experiences itching or redness of skin?	Report symptoms to physician.
	Suggest baking soda or cornstarch baths.
	Discourage use of colognes, shaving lotions, perfumed soaps.
	Encourage use of hypo-allergenic soaps and toiletries.
16) the patient's drug therapy includes a monoamineoxidase inhibitor such as Nardil, Marplan or Niamid?	Instruct the patient regarding diet.
	Eliminate the following foods: chicken livers, aged or natural cheeses, pickled herrings, yeast extract, broad beans.
	Limit intake of coffee, tea, or cola beverages.
	Eliminate beer and wine.
	Observe for hypertensive crisis.
	Caution the patient to avoid taking any medication not prescribed by his physician including over-the-counter drugs such as aspirin, Dristan, cough syrups, and weight reduction pills.
17) the patient's chemotherapy includes lithium carbonate?	Observe the patient for signs of excessive voiding or extreme thirst.
	Force fluids.
	Provide a high caloric diet.
	Report symptoms to physician.
	Monitor lithium levels in blood.
18) the patient is going home on medications?	Emphasize the importance of taking medications as scheduled.
	Provide the patient with written instructions including a list of drugs, time each is taken and special precautions required with each.
	Remind the patient to immediately report any changes in his physical or emotional states and any headache, palpitations, tremulousness, crying or lethargy.
	Remind the patient to continue special dietary modifications.
	Remind the patient to avoid driving a car, using hazardous equipment or machinery, engaging in strenuous exercises and drinking alcoholic beverages.

TABLE 18-2 (continued)	
STUMBLING BLOCKS	**STEPPING STONES**
"What if—	*Try this—*
	Inform the family of special instructions given to patient.
	Set up next appointment to re-evaluate the patient's response to drug therapy and to reinforce and clarify instructions.

activity therapy

Activity therapy is a necessary and vital treatment which provides the individual with opportunities for personal, interpersonal and intrapersonal interaction and growth. Activity therapy is a broad term which encompasses occupational therapy, recreational therapy, educational therapy, industrial therapy, manual arts therapy and gymnastics. Within residential facilities these are usually adjunctive treatments to chemotherapy and psychotherapy. This type of therapy expands an individual's social, recreational, physical, occupational and leisure-time skills. It brings out talents and lets the individual feel proud of his achievements. There are suitable activities for everyone.

Activity therapy is used to promote recovery through the release of excess energy and regression; the provision of a vehicle for self-expression; the practice of social skills in a protected, accepting environment; the acquiring of new knowledge; the development of new technical and creative skills; the correction of physical and psychological impairment; the achievement of self-actualization and the development of a sense of responsibility. Activity therapy is not used merely to occupy the patient's time. It is as important as any other part of the treatment program. Therefore, the nurse's approach should be firm, patient, persistent, observant and helpful. To achieve this approach and to convey to the patient the importance activity therapy plays in his total treatment program, the nurse must demonstrate the attitudes of personal worth, involvement and advocacy.

Specific interventions designed to assist patients who are participating in activity therapy are listed in Table 18-3.

TABLE 18-3
ACTIVITY THERAPY—INTERVENTION AND RATIONALE

Intervention	*Rationale*
Acquire knowledge about kinds of activities available.	to be able to select the appropriate activity for the patient
Assess the patient's emotional and physical needs.	to be able to plan nursing intervention and to demonstrate personal interest in the patient

TABLE 18-3 (continued)

Intervention	Rationale
Assess strengths and weaknesses through interviewing and determine old interests, areas of success and possible areas for developing new interests.	to devise an individualized plan which supports the patient, decreases his level of anxiety, reduces stress and promotes the possibility of successful involvement
Collaborate with colleagues.	to share information, provide consistency and to secure cooperation in devising an effective therapeutic plan
Plan activity schedule and allow for free time.	to prevent exhaustion and to demonstrate the concept of a balance between work, rest and play
Discuss activity schedule with the patient.	to provide information to the patient and create an opportunity for patient input, to maintain a bond of trust and to involve the patient in the decision making process
Elicit the patient's thoughts and feelings regarding his schedule.	to demonstrate acceptance and understanding and to facilitate the clarification of misinterpretations
Encourage the patient to make choices in terms of activities offered.	to assist him to take responsibility for involvement in his own therapeutic regimen
Provide the patient with a copy of his schedule.	to decrease confusion and guard against manipulation and resistance
Indicate firm expectation of adherence to schedule.	to demonstrate care and concern for the patient and to foster his sense of responsibility
Accompany the patient to activity therapies.	to provide security and support, to alleviate anxiety and fear and to convey interest and concern
Stay with the patient for the first few sessions.	to assist the patient in adjusting to a new environment and to observe his initial response to activities and people
Plan and schedule progress conferences with the therapists involved.	to promote collaborative effort on behalf of the patient and to maintain the highest level of effectiveness for the treatment regime
Plan for additional visits and make periodic observations of patient's involvement and responses during activity programs.	to gather information for assessing the patient's progress and to demonstrate sustained interest and concern in his progress
Discuss progress with the patient.	to provide feedback, to give merited praise and to elicit patient's evaluation of self
Revise schedule based on progress reports and patient's input.	to adjust activity therapy to the changing needs of patient

electro-convulsive therapy

Electro-convulsive therapy is a form of shock therapy used to interrupt a patient's current maladaptive pattern of thinking, feeling and behaving. It is an adjunctive somatic treatment that is most commonly utilized for those patients experiencing severe depression, excitation, agitation or for those who are actively suicidal. In essence the procedure is undertaken to produce emotional regression of the patient in time, thereby bringing about modification of the patient's behavior. The treatment is considered effective if the patient begins to evidence a feeling of well-being, ceases to be preoccupied with morbid ideation or is free from agitation. The outcome of this form of treatment permits the individual to be more accessible to others; he demonstrates readiness to socialization and ability to engage in intensive psychotherapy.

In electro-convulsive therapy, nursing intervention is divided into three areas of concern: preparation of the patient prior to the procedure; care of the patient during the procedure; and care of the patient immediately after the procedure. A quiet, firm, confident, nonthreatening approach contributes to the development of a therapeutic atmosphere. The attitudes needed by the nurse to successfully implement such an approach are those of involvement, hopefulness and advocacy.

Specific interventions designed to assist patients undergoing electro-convulsive therapy are listed in Table 18-4.

TABLE 18-4
ELECTRO-CONVULSIVE THERAPY—INTERVENTION AND RATIONALE

Intervention	Rationale
Preparation	
Explain the treatments to the patient in simple, clear, concise terms.	to provide information, to prevent misinterpretation and to alleviate the patient's anxiety
Prepare the patient for and carry out pretreatment workup: assist with the physical examination; check and verify completion of x-rays, EKG and EEG; and secure written consent of the patient or guardian.	to assist in the gathering of clinical data, to safeguard the patient, to protect the patient's rights and to provide legal protection for the treatment team and the hospital
Schedule the treatment and inform the patient of the time, place and frequency.	to implement the therapeutic prescription and to decrease the possibility of additional anxiety
Procure, set up and maintain treatment supplies and equipment: oxygen, carbon dioxide, resuscitator, airway, tracheotomy tray, emergency medication tray, I.V. standard and parenteral fluids, treatment machine, saline solution or electrode jelly, electrodes, headband, mouth gag, tourniquet, syringes, needles, Brevital and Anectine.	to prepare the treatment area for the safe and efficient administration of therapy

TABLE 18-4 (continued)

Intervention	Rationale
Preparation	
Keep the patient NPO for at least four hours prior to treatment.	to prevent aspiration during therapy
Administer prescribed dose of atropine sulfate.	to decrease secretions
Assist the patient to remove all metal objects such as hairpins, watch, rings, medals or other jewelry, glasses, dentures or other prosthetic devices.	to promote safety and prevent injury
Remind the patient to void.	to prevent possibility of rupture of bladder and to prevent incontinence, thereby saving the patient from social embarrassment
Stay with the patient; listen to and closely observe for expressions of anxiety, fear, resistive or manipulative behavior.	to promote psychological comfort through the alleviation of fear and anxiety
Encourage the patient to identify and discuss his feelings about the therapy.	to provide support, to give assurance, to promote comfort and to convey the nurse's acceptance and understanding
Administration	
Accompany the patient to the treatment room.	to provide security, support and reassurance
Proceed with implementation of procedure: instruct the patient to lie supine assisting if necessary; remove shoes; loosen restrictive clothing; recheck for metal objects or dentures; assist in the administration of the Brevital and Anectine; apply conductor to temple area; secure headband in place; insert airway; hyperextend neck; hold jaw in place; assume position needed to apply soft restraint to extremities; advise physician of the patient's and team's readiness.	to prepare the patient for the administration of the treatment and to decrease the patient's level of anxiety
Observe the patient for grand mal seizures, changes in color, and restoration of spontaneous inhalation.	to observe patient's response to treatment and to be ready to institute emergency measures if necessary
Cleanse temple areas.	to prevent irritation to skin
Turn patient on his side.	to prevent patient airway and prevent aspiration
Check for patency of airway.	to insure maintenance of respiration
Raise side rails.	to protect the patient
Remove the patient to recovery room.	to allow time for anesthetic to wear off to provide continuous monitoring of patient's condition

TABLE 18-4 (continued)

Intervention	Rationale
Recovery	
Check pulse and respiration periodically and observe for changes in their rate and in the color of patient.	to assess physiological functioning and to provide data for emergency intervention
Allow patient to sleep until effect of anesthetic has worn off.	to allow for individual differences in reaction time based on individual physiological response or amount of drug given
Reorient the patient to reality as his level of consciousness increases.	to promote patient's feeling of security, to minimize disorientation and confusion and to provide reassurance
Ease the patient to a sitting position on the side of his bed.	to allow for re-establishment of equilibrium
Assist the patient with personal appearance by dressing or rearranging clothing, combing hair and returning personal effects.	to convey personal interest, to minimize anxiety and to promote psychological comfort
Serve meal and assist, if needed.	to meet nutritional needs
Listen to the patient for expressions of physical complaints such as; headache, pain, muscle soreness, dizziness, memory deficits or misinterpretations of treatment or procedure.	to gather information for future interventions, to provide reassurance and to convey interest, acceptance and concern
Complete treatment record form.	to provide information regarding patient's response to treatment
Encourage the patient to participate in his regularly scheduled activities.	to de-emphasize preoccupation with ECT and to emphasize the patient's need for involvement in his total treatment program

suggested readings

Ayd, Frank J. "The Chemical Assault on Mental Illness: The Major Tranquilizers." *American Journal of Nursing,* Vol. 65 No. 4 (April, 1965), 70-78.

————. "The Minor Tranquilizers." *American Journal of Nursing,* Vol. 65 No. 5 (May, 1965), 89-94.

————. "The Anti Depressants." *American Journal of Nursing,* Vol. 65 No. 6 (June, 1965), 78-84.

Beavers, Stacie V. "Music Therapy." *American Journal of Nursing,* Vol. 69 No. 1 (January, 1969), 89.

Cavers, Annie, and Williams, Robert. "The Budget Plan (Behavior Modification for Long-Term Patients)." *Perspectives in Psychiatric Care,* Vol. 9 No. 1 (1971), 13-16.

Cohen, Roberta, "EST and Group Therapy—Improved Care." *American Journal of Nursing,* Vol. 71 No. 6 (June, 1971), 1195-1198.

Gordon, Marjory. "Assessing Activity Tolerance." *American Journal of Nursing,* Vol. 76 No. 1 (January, 1976), 72-75.

Govani, Laura E., and Hayes, Janice E. *Drugs and Nursing Implications.* 2d ed. Appleton-Century-Crofts: New York, 1971.

Kline, Nathan S., and Davis, John M. "Psychotropic Drugs." *American Journal of Nursing,* Vol. 73 No. 1 (January, 1973), 54-62.

Morgan, Arthur James. "Minor Tranquilizers, Hypnotics and Sedatives." *American Journal of Nursing,* Vol. 73 No. 1 (July, 1973), 1220-1222.

Rodman, Morton J., and Smith, Dorothy W. *Pharmacology and Drug Therapy in Nursing.* J. B. Lippincott Co.: Philadelphia, 1968.

chapter 19

planning effective nursing care: rules of thumb

learning objectives

On completion of this chapter the reader should be able to:

1 Define a *nursing care plan*.
2 Describe the scope and use of the nursing care plan.
3 Identify the "rules of thumb" in developing an efficient and effective nursing care plan.
4 Apply the information contained in the nursing care plan to develop nursing interventions.
5 Write an effective nursing care plan based on the nursing process incorporating the identified rules.

Students tend to feel overwhelmed when they are confronted with the task of reading a patient's history, deciding which portions are relevant and from this develop a nursing care plan. Another task they seem to find difficult is the completion of a thoughtful, organized assessment. Although current nursing practice emphasizes the importance of assessment, students and inexperienced practitioners sometimes feel baffled about how to do an assessment. A third major task students and beginning practitioners must cope with is forming therapeutic relationships by establishing and maintaining communication with assigned patients.

To complete a dynamic nursing care plan time, involvement, judgment and coordination are necessary. Time—to observe the patient, interact with him, confer with colleagues, review initial admission information and keep abreast of progress. Involvement—to implement the assessment process, evaluate planned interventions and develop new strategies based on changing needs of the patient. Coordination—to maximize the effectiveness of the health team and to act on the readiness displayed by the patient and the willingness to reorganize the team efforts. Judgment—to be aware of the patient's ability to be involved, recognize the level of patient functioning, be able to intervene at that level and establish and rank priorities.

When confronted with developing a nursing care plan for patients with differing diagnoses, students appear surprised and then disconcerted because the overall goals for care appear to be repetitious. For example, helping the patient to develop a realistic and positive self-concept can apply to both the patient with an anxiety reaction and the patient with schizophrenia. This repetition occurs because all people operate under the same basic human need system. The uniqueness of the care plan evolves as the nurse completes her assessment, identifies the degree to which needs are not being met, identifies the priorities that exist for the particular patient and determines an approach to assist the patient toward optimal functioning.

The setting of realistic objectives for patient care depends on two factors—the extent of the problem and the capacity of the individual to move toward healthy adjustment. In other words, goals for nursing care do not change but the emphasis, approach and intervention does.

Some of the broad nursing care goals which are applicable to all patients in distress, regardless of diagnostic category or practice setting are:

1 To prepare the individual and his family for a hospital experience which meets their needs.

2 To create and maintain an environment which reflects an attitude of honesty, support and genuine concern for patient needs.

3 To help the patient attain and maintain his optimal physical health and mental stability.

4 To help the patient develop a realistic and positive self-concept from which healthy feelings of self-esteem and self-respect can emerge.

5 To increase feelings of security through a climate which demonstrates acceptance of the individual and fosters a feeling of belonging.

6 To cultivate and support an atmosphere which makes use of the individual's assets and encourages him to maximize his potential for change.

7 To identify, explore and demonstrate to the individual satisfactory and effective ways of establishing and maintaining interpersonal relationships.

8 To assist the patient by recognizing the degree of anxiety, frustration and stress he experiences and by providing him with oppor-

tunities to learn effective problem solving methods to deal with crises.

9 To assist the patient to set realistic goals which result in gratification and enable him to function to the level of independence his potential capabilities permit.

10 To develop the concept that life is appreciated and enjoyed through self-directed behavior and that an individual is responsible for maintaining self-directed behavior not only in personal and interpersonal situations, but also in work and leisure activities.

11 To provide continuing support, reassurance and teaching to the patient and his family.

12 To prepare the patient and his family to make the transition from the hospital environment to the community.

Often when a student or a new practitioner enters a psychiatric practice setting for the first time, her anxiety increases. As a result, the nurse sometimes displays an inability to identify patient problems, apply principles and develop methods that result in the effective delivery of competent, qualified nursing care. Frequently, they ask questions like: "Now that I'm here, what do I do?"; "How do I find out?"; and "How do I go about it?" In order to respond to these and similar questions and to assist the student to make the transition from a general practice setting to a psychiatric practice setting, we remind the nurse that psychiatric nursing like all other kinds of nursing care requires order and the setting of priorities. To achieve this end, the nurse must develop a knowledgeable and functional nursing care plan.

a nursing care plan: what is it? what does it do?

A *nursing care plan* is a written outline, a logical orderly, systematized assessment and identification of the patient's problems, objectives for care and the methods and strategies for achieving these objectives. A nursing care plan enables the nurse to establish order, set priorities and develop goals.

TABLE 19-1
NURSING CARE PLAN—DEFINITION AND PURPOSE

What is it?	*What does it do?*
1) A means of individualizing care.	Allows the nurse to adapt basic nursing interventions. Promotes flexibility in accordance with the unique response from each patient within the context of his total experience.
2) A mechanism to assist the patient to solve his problems.	Provides the patient with the opportunity to actively participate in the planning and implementation of his own care.

TABLE 19-1 (continued)

What is it?	What does it do?
3) A mechanism for systematic communication.	Provides to those who will administer the actual care specific, necessary and detailed information. Promotes consistency and continuity of care. Provides a safeguard against a possible breakdown in communication among staff members.
4) A tool for assisting in the coordination of total patient care.	Allows the nurse to plan and collaborate with colleagues and those in other disciplines.
5) A basis for the evaluation of patient care.	Provides the nurse with a point of reference in determining whether or not the expected outcomes were achieved. Identifies the degree to which the plan was effective, thereby creating a basis for realistic, deliberative change.

rules of thumb

To formulate a workable and effective nursing care plan there are rules of thumb which should be considered fundamental to its development. *The first rule of thumb is that the nurse is obliged to make nursing assessments.* This means that a nursing assessment becomes mandatory because assessment is the baseline from which patient problems can be identified. *Nursing assessment* is a process whereby the nurse examines the patient in his totality in an effort to determine the significance, importance or value of subjective and objective data that has been collected regarding the patient and his condition. It involves interviews, observation, evaluation and judgment. In this process, the nurse analyzes all available material such as the patient's history, physical, social and psychological findings, laboratory reports and contributions from other disciplines in order to sort out those factors which seem to have relevance for a given problem and/or need. Assessment provides the nurse with basic information with regard to the patient's 1) life style, 2) physical care needs, 3) emotional needs, 4) need for education and 5) health care goals.

The second rule of thumb is that the nurse must use problem solving as a prerequisite for patient care. Problem solving consists of the identification of a problem, the orderly collection and examination of data related to the problem, the formulation of one or more possible solutions, the implementation of a selected solution and the evaluation of the results. It is a practical, efficient and effective tool. Its use as a method of operation has to become so routine that it is second nature for the nurse to use it as an effective method of intervention on behalf of the patient. Its major benefit to the nurse is that it helps to create objectivity because it provides a method by which the nurse can organize the information she has about the patient as well as identify that information which she still needs to obtain.

The third rule of thumb is that the nurse must write out the nursing care plan. Nursing assessment and problem solving have little impact on patient care until they become a written reality. The written nursing care plan is a basic form of communication concerning the care of the patient. Satisfactory, efficient and relevant nursing care cannot be provided unless those assigned and held accountable for that care know what to do, when to do it, who is to do it and what are the expected results. It also permits the nurse to evaluate her approach and allows her to introduce the necessary modifications to the original plan as the focus of the patient's problem changes. A written nursing care plan provides for three important factors in patient care—consistency, continuity and coordination. Thus, the written nursing care plan provides the nurse and all other staff members with a point of reference.

The fourth rule of thumb is that the nurse must use the nursing care plan as an effective means of communication. The nurse facilitates communication by keeping the lines of communication open and by seeking clarification of that which is communicated. Effective communication requests that the nurse becomes proficient in the use of communication skills, both oral and written. Communication techniques are one of the primary tools of the psychiatric-mental health nurse. These tools enable her to identify assessment factors, use the problem solving approach, write a clear, concise nursing care plan, collaborate with colleagues and other members of the health team and allow the patient to feel and to know that he is of prime concern.

This leads to the _fifth important rule which is the nurse's obligation to preserve the patient's right to privileged communication._ This rule means that the nurse takes all necessary measures to provide for confidentiality. These measures apply to records and recordkeeping, to written and verbal communication, and to the selection of the appropriate place and time to convey to other members of the health team private information about the patient. The nurse has a moral and ethical responsibility to insure that what the patient reveals to her is handled in a professional manner. Consent from the patient must be secured verbally and/or in writing before any information can be shared. It also means that nurses can not exclude the patient from pertinent information concerning himself. The patient has a right to know such things as his temperature, test results, the names of medications prescribed for him and treatment procedures to which he is being subjected. Currently there is much in the literature regarding the rights of patients. And, in fact, the importance of safeguarding patients' rights has resulted in a national movement that has sponsored legislation and a revision of probate court actions in many states. For the patient to provide an "informed consent," he must have basic knowledge of what the treatment entails and the expected outcome of that treatment. The patient has the right of access to any and all records that are kept on him. No one else but those immediately involved with health care delivery to him have the right of access to such information. The emphasis placed on confidentiality and the patient's right of access to information neither automatically absolves the nurse from exercising professional, ethical judgment regarding the amount and depth of information to be provided or withheld, nor does this mean that the nurse is permitted the "right" to make arbitrary choices.

Our *sixth rule of thumb is that the nurse must report in a clear, concise, objective manner.* In the reporting process, the nurse assumes a liaison role between the patient and other care providers. As such, the nurse transmits significant information regarding the appearance, behavior and conversation of the patient. This information adds to the existing data base and serves as another mechanism for continuing systematic communication among members of the health team. The report should contain only that information which is absolutely necessary for the ongoing care of the patient. In order to achieve this type of reporting, extraneous material such as personal opinions, value judgments, hypothetical speculations and irrelevant, subjective comments must be eliminated. One benefit of objective reporting is that it enhances patient care because it facilitates nursing assessment and problem solving. This facilitation is achieved because the mind of the reader or listener is free to look at the problem or situation without the introduction of subjective bias.

Rule seven is that the nurse must engage in peer-group review. Peer-group review is a process in which the individual nurse along with her colleagues assesses and evaluates the quality of care that has been provided a particular patient. This review should be carried out according to established hospital criteria and the official American Nurses Association Standards of Practice. The expected outcome of peer group review is twofold: 1) assistance to the nurse is improving her practice and 2) holding her accountable for that practice. Both of these outcomes insure that the patient is the recipient of the best possible care.

The eighth rule of thumb is that the nurse is obliged to develop, exercise and maintain standards of care. The standards of care we refer to are those standards of practice developed by the Congress for Nursing Practice of the American Nurses Association. Everyone is not required to carry out procedures in an identical manner; but everyone is required to safeguard and adhere to the scientific principles on which the procedures are based. In addition, these standards require that the nurse not short change the patient and his care because of time, load, money or expediency. It means that the nurse takes time with the patient, relates to the patient in such a way so that he does not feel he is a burden or that his needs are less important than those of the patient across the hall. Adherence to standards for care manifests the nurse's appreciation for the very substance of the dignity and worth of mankind and also expresses the nurse's accountability for the delivery of effective patient care.

Rule number nine is that the nurse must collaborate. Collaboration means the nurse actively seeks to share her knowledge and expertise. It implies that the nurse acknowledges and seeks to include the expertise peculiar to other members of the health team in carrying out the total treatment program of the patient. It means that the nurse volunteers information about the patient's progress and concerns to those of the appropriate disci-

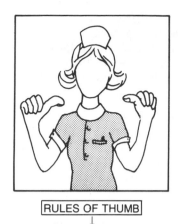

RULES OF THUMB
↓
1. Make Nursing Assessments
↓
2. Use Problem Solving
↓
3. Write Out Nursing Care Plan
↓
4. Use Nursing Care Plan for Communication
↓
5. Preserve Privileged Communication
↓
6. Report Clearly, Concisely and Objectively
↓
7. Engage in Peer Group Review
↓
8. Maintain Standards of Care
↓
9. Seek Collaboration

Figure 19-1

plines. Collaboration benefits the nurse in that it allows her to seek consultation for the purpose of clarification and validation of her own nursing observations, assessments and interventions.

As stated in the beginning of this chapter, all nursing care requires order and priority setting. These rules of thumb are general prerequisites the nurse needs in order to develop order and to set priorities in planning a sound, practical approach to the implementation of effective nursing care. Again, we re-emphasize that there are some approaches and nursing care practices which cut across all fields of practice and that each specialty area of practice must also operate on these. The uniqueness found in each specialty results primarily from the specific area of focus and the manifested needs of the patient. The constant is the framework, the nursing process, and the principles which govern its implementation and operation. What varies is the presenting problems of the patient, the major symptoms associated with the problem, specific methods of intervention available and the way in which the nurse implements and utilizes the potential of the creative therapeutic self.

This chapter points out some very specific information that the nurse needs to have in order to carry out an operational nursing care plan. We have identified nine rules of thumb for this purpose.

In Chapter 21 these "rules of thumb" are applied in detail by in what we consider an optimal, effective and meaningful nursing care plan.

suggested readings

Beyers, Marjorie, and Phillips, Carol. "Keys to Successful Leadership." *Nursing '74,* Vol. 4 No. 7 (July, 1974), 51-58.

Burton, Genevieve. *Personal, Impersonal and Interpersonal Relations.* Springer: New York, 1964.

Byers, Virginia B. *Nursing Observation.* Wm. C. Brown Co.: Dubuque, Iowa, 1973.

Carrieri, Virginia Kohlman, and Sitzman, Judith. "Components of the Nursing Process." *Nursing Clinics of North America,* Vol. 6 No. 1 (March, 1971), 115-124.

Dolan, Marion B. "Shelly Was Angry—So Was The Staff." *Nursing '74,* Vol. 4 No. 6 (June, 1974), 86-88.

Jacobson, Sylvia R. "A Study of Interpersonal Collaboration." *Nursing Outlook,* Vol. 22 No. 12 (December, 1974), 751-755.

Joel, Lucille A., and Davis, Shirley M. "A Proposal for Base Line Data Collection for Psychiatric Care." *Perspectives In Psychiatric Care,* Vol. II No. 2 (1973), 48-58.

Kron, Thora. *Communication in Nursing.* W. B. Saunders Co.: Philadelphia, 1967.

Marrimer, Ann. *The Nursing Process: A Scientific Approach to Nursing Care.* C. V. Mosby Co.: St. Louis, 1975.

Mayers, Marlene. *A Systematic Approach to the Nursing Care Plan.* Appleton-Century-Crofts: New York, 1976.

McCain, R. Faye. "Nursing by Assessment—Not Intuition." *American Journal of Nursing,* Vol. 65 No. 4 (April, 1965), 82-84.

Mundiger, Mary O'Neill, and Jouron, Grace Dotterer. "Developing a Nursing Diagnosis." *Nursing Outlook,* Vol. 23 No. 2 (February, 1975), 94-98.

Naugle, Ethel H. "The Differences Caring Makes." *American Journal of Nursing,* Vol. 73 No. II (November, 1973), 1890-1891.

Roy, Sister Collecta. "A Diagnostic Classification System for Nursing." *Nursing Outlook,* Vol. 23 No. 2 (February, 1975), 90-94.

Standards: Psychiatric Mental Health Nursing Practice. American Nurses Association: Kansas City, Missouri, 1973.

part 4

chapter 20

a case presentation: mrs. sheila franklin

learning objectives

On completion of this chapter the reader should be able to:

1 Identify relevant social data.
2 Understand the relationship of social data to the formation of dysfunction.
3 Identify specific symptomotology from the social data base.
4 Integrate the psychosocial dynamics as they relate to the developmental process, the effects of stress and crisis and the sequence of pathology.

The following narrative demonstrates how pathology develops in a life and is then identified from a case history. The pathological characteristics of schizophrenia are pointed out as well as the socio-psychological and physiological factors particular to an individual patient.

Mrs. Sheila Franklin, a 30-year-old, widowed, Caucasian female is the mother of an 8-year-old daughter, Debby.

family history

Mrs. Franklin's father, William J. Mitchell, a professional golfer and musician, is a quiet, timid person. Her mother, Mary Rose, is strict and controlling and makes all the rules for the family. Mrs. Franklin is one of three children. She has a married sister, Evelyn James, 32 years old, who had a "nervous breakdown" after the birth of her first child ten years ago, and a brother, Thomas Mitchell, aged 20, who is unmarried and lives at home.

> Family history reveals the familiar pattern found in histories of schizophrenic patients—domineering mother, passive father.

developmental history

As a child, Mrs. Franklin was quiet and obedient. Her mother said she was a "good little girl" who never got into trouble. She seldom needed discipline but was content to sit on the floor and play with her dolls. Her teachers considered her a good student except they wished she would "talk a little more and look out the window less." During her high school years she liked to read and never complained about her school work. She made friends easily but established no close relationships. She was considered a "loner." In her junior year she began having occasional dates with Paul Franklin, a college student whom Sheila had known all her life. She refused to join in school social activities because she "needed the time to 'bone up' on math and sciences" since she planned to enter nursing school after graduation.

> "Good" behavior during early childhood is used to gain approval from adults. Playing alone, talking little and gazing out of the window might be considered as early manifestations of autistic behavior. The pattern of withdrawal appears to become more pronounced during high school years.

Sheila was accepted into a school of nursing. After six months, she contracted infectious mononucleosis. During convalescence she decided that she was no longer interested in nursing and that she would leave school to get her trousseau ready for her forthcoming marriage with Paul Franklin. She made plans, placed orders for clothes and household articles and was very much involved in the total preparation for the wedding. However, she failed to keep appointments for fittings and alterations; she scheduled two appointments for the same time and as a result her mother and fiance completed most of the transactions she started. The night before the wedding, she paced her room for two hours, packed and unpacked her suitcase three times and finally insisted on telling her parents all the factors which indicated to her that she was definitely ready for marriage.

> Increased levels of anxiety interfere with the completion of projects begun and give rise to feelings of insecurity and self-doubt as evidenced by indecisiveness and vacillation.

In the first two months of her marriage, she seemed to enjoy taking care of the apartment, shopping and learning to cook the things her husband liked. She and her husband visited her parents on occasion but she was reluctant to invite anyone in or to go out. She stated that she felt uncomfortable at the home of her in-laws; she felt sure they thought she was not good enough for Paul. She began to complain of being tired and used this complaint to reject Paul's sexual advances. As the months passed she slept later than usual and found it more difficult to care for the apartment and herself. She took to wearing her pajamas and housecoat all day. This change in behavior concerned her husband and he insisted that she have a physical examination which revealed that she was about three months pregnant. Upon learning of the pregnancy, Paul immediately assumed many of the usual household routines that she had previously neglected.

> Apathy is demonstrated by a loss of interest in her surroundings and lack of attention to her physical appearance. These two behaviors also indicate early signs of regressive behavior.

Before the baby was born, her husband left on a business trip and was killed in an airplane accident. Mrs. Franklin accepted the news of her husband's death calmly but after the funeral she again complained of tiredness and frequently missed appointments at the prenatal clinic saying she forgot or "there was no need to go." Her mother said that during this period she never cried, just sat in the rocker, continuously rocking back and forth staring out of the window.

> Emotional detachment and withdrawal are becoming more pronounced. In addition, symptoms of rationalization and denial are beginning to appear.

After the baby was born Mrs. Franklin said that she was happy that the baby was a little girl. But she expressed fear about caring for her. She told her mother that she thought she might drop or hurt the baby in some way. One day Mrs. Franklin was observed bending over the baby's crib, gently stroking the baby's arm. Suddenly, she squeezed Debby's hand until the infant started to cry.

> This behavior toward the child displays marked ambivalence toward herself and motherhood.

After this incident she ran out of the room, left the house and was gone for two hours. Her brother found her sitting on a park bench several blocks from home. As soon as she saw him, she asked if he came to tell her that Paul was home. Without waiting for him to respond she continued, "If only he would come back, I know Mom and Dad did not want us to get married but we did, I should be living with him—not at home with them. Why are they keeping me away from him? Debby needs a father. Oh! Why am I sitting here for, I have so much to do, the baby must be hungry . . . it's too nice a day to work, the sun feels good . . . warm and bright but I feel cold and alone. . . ."

> This segment of social history demonstrates autistic thinking as indicated by her belief that Paul was still alive. The stream of thought begins to show the looseness of association and confabulation. However, this is the

first indication of it and it is still minimal. Another symptom displayed is that of loneliness and possible feelings of isolation.

Mrs. Franklin's parents and her obstetrician were able to convince her that she should seek psychiatric help. She was placed on an antipsychotic medication and saw a psychiatrist each week for six months. She made continuous progress and was discharged after this six-month period.

Mrs. Franklin enrolled in a secretarial school, completed the course of study and obtained a job in an office which she held for five years. She and Debby lived with her parents. Mrs. Franklin helped her mother, assumed some of the ordinary household expenses and managed to devote a great deal of time to her daughter, especially on weekends. She seldom dated, said she compared all men to Paul and they just didn't measure up. She received three pay raises at the office, expressed satisfaction with the job, and never had any complaints about the work.

One day about a year ago she came home from work and suddenly announced to her family that she and Debby were moving to Arizona to live near her sister. She said she was unhappy at work: "The other girls leave me the hardest and most complicated assignments and they blame me for the mistakes in the files. Now they don't like the color of my clothes—my blouse would be prettier if it was yellow instead of blue. I'm getting tired of their checking up on me, always asking, 'Did you do this—did you finish that job—will you type this for me.' I finally said no, I cleared out my desk and quit."

> Sudden onset of suspiciousness, ideas of reference, delusional ideation, and impulsiveness may be indicative of psychopathology.

Evelyn James, Mrs. Franklin's sister was glad to have her come to Arizona and promised to help her find a job and an apartment. Meanwhile, she and Debby could live with them. Mrs. Franklin got along well with Evelyn—they made up for lost time since they hadn't seen each other for at least four years. Evelyn and her children had fun showing Sheila and Debby around the city. They toured various sections so that Mrs. Franklin could decide where she'd like to live. The sisters shared the work at home. Mrs. Franklin studied the daily newspaper ads and made lists of people to contact both for an apartment and for a job interview. After six months there was still no job nor had she found a place to live. When Mrs. James tried to discuss the situation with her, Sheila offered numerous reasons why the apartments were unsuitable. As for the job interviews, she gave multiple reasons why none of the positions were acceptable: they wanted to know too much about her personal life; one employer expected too much for the money he was paying; one placement was like the job she just left—too many girls in the office and she would be the newest employee and therefore they would soon take advantage of her.

> Excuses indicate excessive use of rationalization and projection. This behavior also demonstrates her passive dependency.

Mrs. James tried to be understanding and reassuring, and told Sheila to keep looking until she found something more to her satisfaction. At the end of another month, Evelyn tried again to discuss the situation. Sheila began to cry, insisting she was trying but there was really very little available. If she and Debby were creating financial problems for the James' she could pay board; it wouldn't take long to transfer the money from her savings account. A few more weeks passed, this time both Mr. and Mrs. James talked with Mrs. Franklin. She listened for awhile, then in an angry tone blurted out that it was clear to her that they really did not care about her and she certainly would not stay where she was not wanted. She abruptly left the living room, helped Debby get settled into bed and immediately started packing. The next day she bought bus tickets for herself and Debby and returned to Cleveland.

Pressure from family precipitated an increase in irrational behavior in the form of impulsiveness, hostility and reappearance of ideas of persecution.

Her parents met them at the bus station. On the way home, she told her parents that they were no longer welcome in Arizona. Evelyn bossed Debby around and her kids made trouble, caused fights and then blamed Debby for them. Debby said, "No! Mommy! No!, Aunt Evelyn was nice to me and I liked Jimmy and Janey and Susie." Mrs. Franklin told her, "Shush," and said she certainly knew better than a little girl what was really going on. Sheila then proceeded to relate to her parents how Evelyn had grown jealous of her, interfered with her getting any of "those good jobs" and prevented her from renting "wonderful apartments." The next few days Sheila was illogical, unreasonable and argumentative. Her mother tried to convince her that she should see her former therapist or be admitted to a hospital.

Behavior at this point indicates Sheila is demonstrating increasing deterioration of her thought process. Use of the nebulous "they," the distortion of the situation with her sister and her inability to maintain an objective viewpoint illustrates this increase in her pathology.

Sheila refused, stating, "Everyone seems to think there is something wrong with me. No one considers that anyone else is wrong. As long as I do what you all want then everything is okay, but as soon as I say no, it's a different story. Nobody cares when I am being pushed around but as soon as I complain then there is something wrong with me!"

Her statement is an example of denial, rationalization and projection.

For the next two weeks Sheila kept to her own room except for meals. She ate little, stating she wasn't hungry. She did not talk much but did respond to questions.

There is an increase in her pattern of withdrawal and apathetic behavior. Her behavior also demonstrates negativism, loss of appetite and mutism.

One day during lunch she told her mother that she again dreamed someone tried to kill her and Debby. The mother became frightened after hearing this and the family agreed to make arrangements for an emergency admission for Sheila.

> Her repeated dreams of someone trying to harm her is part of a now well-developed system of persecutory delusions. The dream may indicate the possibility of suicidal and homicidal tendencies.

During the admission procedure Mrs. Franklin was obviously anxious and overtalkative. She told the doctor that she had been fighting strange incidents and plots against her for at least seven years.

> Persecutory delusions have become more pronounced and expansive.

"Everything has been so hard. It would have been different if Paul had lived. People don't pick on women when their husbands are around. Have you any idea what it is like for a mother to bring up a child alone? Debby is a good girl but sometimes she does strange things."

> She has made a transition from one thought to a completely different idea, indicating more pronounced looseness in association. Rationalization is also apparent.

"I did not tell anybody before because they just wouldn't believe me. John, my sister's husband, made improper advances toward me. That's why we came back. I was afraid. What really scared me was all those men on the bus and at the bus station looking at me so funny. Even my own brother; I keep my door locked 'cause you just can't trust anyone these days, not even your own family."

> Denial of normal sexual feelings resulting in projective behavior.

Mrs. Franklin was admitted to a psychiatric unit of a general hospital with an initial diagnosis of schizophrenia, paranoid type.

This social history details and demonstrates the sequence of events that eventuated the necessity for psychiatric hospitalization. It is at this point in time that those nurses who function in the institutional treatment setting begin to implement a realistic, operational nursing care plan to enable Mrs. Franklin and her family to resume their usual daily living experiences.

chapter 21

assessment and nursing care plans for mrs. sheila franklin

learning objectives

On completion of this chapter the reader should be able to:

1 Trace the development of an effective nursing care plan.
2 Extract relevant data that contributes to the assessment and the care of the patient.
3 Identify the application of theory to practice.

Nursing care for any patient begins when the patient enters the door and meets the nurse for the first time. In the initial confrontation with the patient, the nurse begins the assessment process. The nursing care plan that is eventually formulated takes into account the admission procedure and the patient's response to it, the assessment interview, the physical, sociological, and psychological findings as well as the continuous assessment of the patient's response to the care provided. The following is a graphic representation of the hospital experience of Mrs. Sheila Franklin and the actual step-by-step process the nurses used in her care.

admission to the hospital

Miss Maris, R.N., responded to the call from the emergency room and escorted Mrs. Franklin to the ward. Mrs. Franklin acknowledged the introduction of the nurse by nodding her head, but said nothing. Walking down the hall toward the elevator, the nurse observed that Mrs. Franklin avoided walking next to her, looked from side to side and peered intently at any open doorway. As they approached the elevator, Mrs. Franklin said, "You don't expect me to get into that cage!" Miss Maris replied, "This is the elevator, but we could walk up the stairs to the next floor, if you'd rather."

> Mrs. Franklin's behavior demonstrates suspiciousness. There is evidence of an increased level of anxiety, fear and distrust.

On reaching the ward, Miss Maris introduced Mrs. Franklin to the head nurse. Mrs. Franklin looked at her and said, "What do you think you are going to do for me here? There's nothing wrong with me!"

> The repeated use of denial indicates a lack of insight. Mistrust of the physical and personal environment is conveyed through her actions and comments.

Neither of the nurses directly referred to Mrs. Franklin's statements. Miss Maris calmly and with self-assurance said, "Come, I'll take you to your room. I'll show you where to put your things. I will wait for you until you put them away or I'll help you, if you like." After the unpacking was completed, Miss Maris sat down with Mrs. Franklin to explain the admission and other hospital routines and to answer whatever questions she might have. The nurse decided to forego the actual procedures and initial interview because she felt Mrs. Franklin needed time to adapt herself to her new environment.

> This decision was based on the assessments the nurse had already made regarding Mrs. Franklin's level of anxiety and degree of suspiciousness.

The nurse kept her explanations short and to the point and briefly answered questions asked by the patient. In less than an hour Mrs. Franklin was ready to leave her room to see the ward and continue with the admission procedures. In the meantime, Miss Maris consulted the ward social worker about the patient's history and planned to continue the assessment interview after lunch.

The following "Assessment—Psychiatric Nursing History" form was completed by Miss Maris.

assessment-psychiatric nursing history

A. Personal Information

Name *Sheila Franklin*   Date of Admission *3/1/*

Date of birth   *5/30/*   Date of Assessment *3/1/*

Age _30_ Sex _F_ Marital Status - Single _____

Married _____

Widowed ___✓___

Divorced _____

Separated _____

National Origin _English - Irish_

Address _1243 Meadowbrook Rd._ Phone _909-1275_

Cleveland, Ohio

Name of Nearest Relative _William J. Mitchell_

Relationship _Father_

Address _(Same as above)_ Phone _909-1275_

Religious Preference _Protestant_

Church Affiliation _St. Paul's Methodist_

Do you want your clergy to visit? _No_

Do you want the hospital chaplain to visit? _No_

Previous Hospitalizations:

Diagnosis	Date
Pregnancy	_1970 69_
_T & A_	_1953_

Medications currently being used:

Name	Dosage
None	

Do you have any known sensitivity to drugs? *No*

Do you have any allergies? *No*

B. Social Functioning

1. Family Constellation:

a. Position and role in family:

Second of three siblings

b. Family Members:

Spouse: Name *Paul Franklin* Age *Deceased*

Parents: Name *Hon. J Mitchell* Age *55*

Name *Mary Rose*   Age *51*

Siblings: Name *Evelyn James*   Age *32*

Name *Thomas Mitchell* Age *20*

Name_____ Age_____

Name_____ Age_____

Children: Name *Debby Franklin* Age *8*

Name_____ Age_____

Name_____ Age_____

Name_____ Age_____

c. Living Arrangements:

Lives with parents, daughter, and unmarried brother in parent's home

d. To whom do you relate to best?

Brother

2. Occupational and Educational Status:

    a. Occupation *Secretary*

    b. Place of Employment *Unemployed*

    c. Date of last employment *Approx. one year ago*

    d. If unemployed, source of income *Social Security - Survivor's Benefits.*

    e. Years of schooling *High school - six month secretarial course*

3. Recreational Activities:

    a. Interests? *Did not respond*

    b. Hobbies? *??*

    c. Membership in Clubs or Organizations? *??*

C. Biophysiological Functioning

    1. Vital Signs: T *98.8* P *86* R *20* BP *124/72*

        a. Signs and symptoms indicating possible deficit:

            None

        b. Nursing intervention required:

2.   Sensory Functions:

    a. Any hearing difficulty?   Yes___ No ✔

       1. Describe:

       2. Hearing Aid: Yes___ No ✔

       3. Provision for batteries_____

    b. Any difficulty seeing?   Yes___ No ✔

       1. Describe:

       2. Wears glasses: For reading____ All Day ____

       3. Has glass eye: Yes___ No ✔

    c. Any other prosthetic devices? *No*

       1. Describe:

       2. Nursing Intervention Required:

    d. Any decreased ability or inability to detect changes in skin temperature? *No*

    e. Any numbness, tingling, dizziness, blurred vision? *No*

    f. Other:

3. Motor Functions:

    a. Physical limitations and disabilities? *No*

    b. Seizures? *No*

4. Personal Hygiene:

    a. Bathing:

        1. Time: A.M._____ P.M. *10*___

        2. Type: Shower_____Tub _✓_Other_____

    b. Care of Teeth:

        1. Dentures   Yes___ No _✓_

        2. Usual cleaning time *Two times a day*

    c. Care of Skin:

        1. Condition: Oily____ Dry _✓_ Moist____

        2. Color: Pale____ Flushed _✓_Jaundiced____

                   Cyanotic_____ Normal_____

        3. Skin is: Broken_____ Bruised___Edematous__

        4. Abnormalities: Rash___ Lesion___Other *Clear*

           a. Describe location and extent:

                          —

           b. Nursing intervention required:

                          —

        5. Do you use anything on your skin at home: *No*

d. Care of Hair:

    1. Length: Average__✓__ Long_____ Short_____

    2. Appearance: Clean_____ Well-groomed_____

                Unkempt__✓__Stringy____Straggly____

    3. Condition: Dry_____ Oily_____ Shiney_____

             Dull__✓__

    4. How often do you wash your hair?__*weekly*__

             Self__✓__

             Beauty shop_____

             Barber shop_____

e. Care of Nails: (Hands and Feet)

    1. Condition: Hard_____ Soft_____ Long_____

             Short__✓__ Average_____

    2. Uses: File_____ Emery Boards_____ Buffer____

           Scissors____ Clippers____ Polish_____

f. Feminine Hygiene: *Evidence of nail biting*

    1. Menstrual Cycle:

        a. Frequency of period__*q 28 days*__

        b. Number of Days__*5*__

        c. Amount of Discharge: Sm___Mod__✓__Heavy___

        d. Type of absorbent protection used:

                Napkins__✓__

                Tampons_____

        e. Date of last menstrual period__*2/27/*__

    2. Birth Control Measures:

        a. Contraceptives: Oral_____ I.U.D._____

        b. Rhythm: Yes_____ No_____

      c. Other: Yes_____No_____ Describe:

      d. None____✓_____

    3. Douching: Yes_____ No__✓_____

      a. Solution_____

      b. Equipment used_____

    4. Hair Removal:

      a. Uses: Depilatory Cream_____ Razor__✓____

      b. Type of razor: Electric_____Safety__✓___

    5. Cosmetics: Yes_✓_ No_____

      a. Uses: Powder__✓____ Perfume____ Lipstick_✓_

                 Deodorant_✓_ Cremes____ Lotions_____

                 Hairspray_____

  g. Masculine Hygiene:

    1. Shaving: Razor: Electric_____Safety_____

    2. Cosmetics: Shaving Creme___Skin Conditioner___

              After Shave Lotion___ Cologne_____

              Hairspray_____

    3. Athletic Support: Yes_____ No_____

5.   Elimination: Usual pattern

  a. Bowels:

    1. Frequency___*daily*_____ Time___*a.m.*_____

    2. Laxative (specify)_____*no*_____

  b. Bladder:

    1. Frequency___*2-3 times*___ Time_*"I don't know"*_

    2. Nocturnal Voiding: Yes_____ No_✓_

c. Any change noted since illness? Diarrhea_____

No

Constipation_____

Incontinence_____

Nocturnal Voiding__

d. Other problems:

1. Colostomy: Yes_____ No__✓__

2. Ileostomy: Yes_____ No__✓__

3. Means of care and regulation:

6.   Sleep and Comfort Pattern:

a. Usual bedtime __11:30 p.m.__

b. Number of hours of sleep __9-10 hours__

"Sometimes I sleep, sometimes I don't, My thoughts keep me awake."

1. Uninterrupted: Yes_____ No__✓__

2. Up during night: Time_____ Frequency_____

c. Accustomed to a single room: Yes__✓__ No_____

d. Nap: Yes_____ No__✓__ Time_____

e. Comfort measures:

1. Pillow: Yes__✓__ No_____ Number __Two__

2. Blanket: Yes__✓__ No_____ Number __One__

3. Night Light:Yes__✓__ No_____

4. Windows: Open_____ Closed __✓__

5. Bedtime Snack: Yes__✓__ No_____ Specify __anythi__

6. Sleeping Pills: Yes_____ No__✓__ Name_____

Dosage_____

Sleeps with room door locked.

7.   Nutritional Pattern:

a. Height *5'6"*   Weight *130*

b. Food Habits:

Meal Pattern	Time	Usual Food
B	$8^{30} - 9^{30}$	juice coffee
L *Skips lunch*		
D	" *when I feel like eating* "	anything
S	*Before bed*	anything

c. Food Likes:

" *I'm not fussy* "

d. Food Dislikes:

" *My mother cooks what I like.* "

e. Food Allergies:

None

f. Religious Restrictions:

None

g. Fluid Habits:

Beverage	Temperature
B *Black coffee*	*hot*
L	
D *coffee - milk*	*hot - cold*
S *juice - pop*	*cold.*

h. Beverage Dislikes:

tea — diet pop

i. Any difficulties with food or fluid intake? *No*

Chewing_____ Swallowing_____ Nausea_____ Vomiting___

Food Appetite_____ Distention_____ Other_____

ɜ. What do you usually do for a stomach upset at home?
"I don't have any — there's nothing wrong c̄ me".
Mother states she chews Rolaids constantly.

D. Mental - Emotional - Behavioral Functioning:

1. Appearance: *On admission :*

a. Facial expressions:

angry __✔__ cheerful_____ disinterested_____

blank _____ frowning __✔__ dissatisfied_____

happy_____ haggard_____ questioning __✔__

worn_____ smiling_____ bewildered_____

sad_____ tearful_____ interested_____

b. Eyes:

open___✔___ sparkling____ staring_____

closed_____ darting___✔___ fixed_____

c. Complexion: healthy_____ sallow_____ pasty_____

ruddy_____ other *slightly flushed*

d. Grooming and Dress:

1. Clothing: clean_____ pressed_____ wrinkled __✔__

ragged_____ soiled_____ burned_____

2. Shoes: Shined_____ Scuffed_____ Worn_____

3. Stockings: Yes_____ No __✔__

4. Socks: Yes_____ No_____

e. Body Language:

  1. Posture: Erect__✓__ Sagging_____

  2. Movement: Normal____ Slow_____ Fast__✓___

              Relaxed_____ Coordinated_____

              Hyperactive_____

	Head	Face	Torso	Extremities
Trembling	____	____	____	____
Twitching	____	____	____	____
Spasms	____	____	____	____
Rocking	____	____	____	____
Immobile	____	____	____	____
Rigid	✓	____	✓	✓
Tics	____	____	____	____

 2. Behavior:

  shy _____   oriented__✓__   impatient__✓__

  bold_____   restless__✓__   attentive_____

  aloof_✓__   euphoric____   suspicious__✓__

  bossy_____   sarcastic_✓__   ritualistic___

  alert_✓__   withdrawn_✓__   distrustful_✓__

  labile____   demanding____   uninhibited____

  fearful_✓__   confident____   disoriented____

  playful___   apathetic____   apprehensive_✓__

  confused__   irritable_✓__   antagonistic___

  agitated___   impulsive____   distractable___

  critical_✓__   seductive____

 3. Communication:

  a. Tone: Soft____ Loud_✓__ Average____ Clipped_✓___

        Whispering____

b. Speech Difficulties: Language Barrier___

   Lisping____ Stuttering____ Other *None*

c. Flow of Speech:

   Talkative _✓_   Mute _____

   Average _____   Guarded_✓_

   Hesitant _____   Mumbles_____

   Constant flow ___   Gregarious, initiating__

   Repetitious _✓_   Quiet, non-initiating__

   Relevant _____   Monosyllables _✓_

   Irrelevant _____

d. Perception and Thinking:

   1. Intellectual Functioning:

      a. Impaired Memory: Yes_____ No _✓_

                          Recent __Remote __

      b. Imparied judmgent:Yes_✓_ No_____

      c. Brief Attention Span: Yes_✓_No_____

      d. Lacks Ability to Concentrate: Yes_✓_No *Appears preoccupied*

      e. Misinterprets: Yes_✓_ No_____

      f. Logical: Yes_____ No_✓_

      g. Ability to Abstract: Yes_____ No_✓_ *See admn notes*

      h. Concrete: Yes_✓_ No_____ *see admission n[o]*

   2. Perception:

      a. Impaired: Yes_✓_ No_____ *perceived elevator "cage".*

      b. Types of Impairment:

         1. Illusions: Yes_✓_ No_____

         2. Hallucinations: Visual__Auditory____

                            Tactile___ Gustatory_____

                            Olfactory_____

3. Other: Describe: *None noted — denied by patient, seemed guarded in response to the question about hearing voices.*

3. Thought Progressions: Normal___ Abnormal ✓

Blocking_____ Flight of Ideas_____

Incoherence____Circumstantiality ✓

Retardation_____

4. Thought Content:

a. Delusions: Somatic____ Ideas of Reference ✓

"People take advantage of me" Grandeur___Persecutory ✓_____

Self-accusatory_____

b. Obsessions: Yes___ No___ Describe:

c. Phobias: Yes___ No___ Describe:

4. Ego Assessment:

a. Defense Mechanisms Used:

Denial ___✓____   Repression _____

Projection ✓___   Regression _____

Rationalization ✓   Suppression _____

Identification ___   Reaction Formation___

Introjection _____   Conversion _____

Displacement _____   Sublimation _____

Undoing _____   Substitution _____

Compensation _____

b. Self-Evaluation:

1. How do you see yourself?

   polite ✓   friendly ✓   easy going ____

   loving ____   likeable ____   trustworthy ____

   honest ✓   reliable ✓   independent ✓

   unkind ____   cautious ____   considerate ____

   selfish ____   dependent ____   short tempered __

2. What is your usual mood? Has it changed?

   "Sometimes I feel sad. I miss my husband."

3. What kinds of things make you feel better/(worse?)

   "When people blame me for things that happen."

4. Is there any time of day in which you think more clearly, do things better or feel best?

   "At night". Wasn't able to give any reason or further explanation.

5. What are some of the things you think and worry about?

   "My little girl — Debby."

6. Does time go quickly or slowly for you?

   "Don't know".

7. Do you find it easy to talk to other people?

   "What do you want to know for?"
   (Before I could respond, answered yes.)

8. What kind of person do you find most interesting?

   "Haven't thought about it —
   someone like my Paul."

9. What do you expect of yourself?

   "To work, to be a good mother,"

   Of family?

   "Leave me alone"! (Sounds angry)

   Of friends?

   "To be friends"

   Of people in general?

   "Not to push me around — to live
   and let live."

10. What were the circumstances which led up to
    your coming to the hospital?

    "My parents think I need to be
    here."

11. Have you ever felt a desire or tried to injure yourself in any way?

No verbal response — moved back in chair — appeared angry.

12. Have you noticed any changes in your sexual interest/functioning?

No verbal response — shook head no.

13. What would you like the nursing staff to help you with while you are in the hospital?

"I don't know."

14. What did you find most helpful/least helpful when you were hospitalized before?

"They had good food."

15. What do you expect to happen to you after your experience in the hospital?

"I don't know — work I suppose and care for Debby 'til she grows up."

E.   Visitors:

   1. Are your friends and family able to visit you?

Yes

   2. Do you want any limitations of visitors? *"Yes,*

I don't want to see my parents.
They put me in here — now they
can stay away!"

NURSING SUMMARY:

1.   What does the patient "want" or need? *Wants: To be left alone.*
     Needs: a. *decreased suspiciousness*   c. *develop trust*
          b. *develop positive relationships*   d. *develop realistic sense of*
                                            responsibility

2.   Is attainment within the realm of the patient's capabi-
     lities and potential?
     Yes — Previous past experience indicates potential.

3.   What prevents the individual from reaching identified
     goals? *Poor self-concept; feelings of inadequacy;*
         guilt re. husband's death; suspiciousness;
         anxiety.

4.   What changes in behavior could result in more productive
     living patterns through health teaching? *Better dietary habits;*
     Organization; priority setting and use of time; Learning to
     cope with feelings of anger, anxiety, guilt and loneliness.

5.   What role does the family play in the individual's pat-
     tern of living? *Parents are very much interested in her*
     welfare but contribute to her dependency. Brother is
     supportive and encouraging.

6.   To what extent can the family be involved in the indivi-
     dual's care? *To a large extent, expressed interest*
     and a willingness to help.

7. What resources are available to the individual and his
    family when he returns to the community?

Mental Health Clinic   *Social groups and*
Family Services   *Church group.*
Job Counseling

initial nursing care plan

After completing the interview, Miss Maris wrote a preliminary care plan based on her conclusions. She then scheduled a total team conference with the ward staff (physician, psychologist, social worker, occupational and recreational therapists, the nursing assistants assigned to her team, the head nurse and herself) and Mrs. Franklin for 10:00 a.m. the next day. The purpose for the conference was to formulate a total treatment program for Mrs. Franklin. The outcome of the ward conference provides the nurse with the necessary information to design a nursing care plan in conjunction with the other nursing staff.

In developing the initial nursing care plan, Miss Maris identified three major nursing care goals:

1 To assist Mrs. Franklin in achieving successful adaptation to the hospital environment.

2 To prepare Mrs. Franklin for involvement in the total treatment plan.

3 To obtain needed information through observation and interaction with Mrs. Franklin in order to facilitate the ongoing development of her nursing care plan.

The initial nursing care plan devised by Miss Maris is shown in Table 21-1.

TABLE 21-1
INITIAL NURSING CARE PLAN

NAME: Sheila Franklin   NURSE: Miss Maris   DATE: 3/1/19___

Nursing Care Goals	Patient Problems	Nursing Intervention	Rationale	Results of Intervention
To help develop a sense of safety and help her to begin to establish rapport with staff.	1) Suspicious: a) Sits facing the door. b) Looks over her shoulder as she walks down the hall. c) Fearful because she cannot lock her room door. 2) Regressive: a) Wishes to stay in her room. b) Refuses to meet other patients.	1) Approach in a calm, self-assured manner. 2) Take time to explain scheduled procedures. Tell her: a) Laboratory technician will take blood samples at 8 a.m. b) She will go to x-ray and EKG at 8:30 a.m. c) Breakfast will be served when she returns to ward. 3) Answer call bell promptly. 4) Make positive approaches several times during evening. a) Invite Mrs. F. to: 1) Watch T.V. 2) Meet other patients. 3) Have a snack.	People displaying symptoms of suspicion, distrust, fear are often threatened by interpersonal relationships; therefore a friendly but reserved approach is more likely to succeed. Opportunities for satisfying relationships and feelings of security are increased when the individual is able to see others as truthful, dependable and capable.	Patient responded to information with: "I hope they are on time—I hate to wait." Refused to come out of her room and said, "Maybe tomorrow."

TABLE 21-1 (continued)

NAME: Sheila Franklin NURSE: Miss Maris DATE: 3/1/19___

Nursing Care Goals	Patient Problems	Nursing Intervention	Rationale	Results of Intervention

		b) Attempt to find out:
		  1) What she usually does with her free time.
		  2) Interests or hobbies, past and present.
		  3) Offer assistance at bedtime:
		    a. Check on need for toilet articles.
		    b. Remind not to drink fluids after midnight.
			Trust and confidence are enhanced by a demonstration of concern and interest.	Responded to all questions briefly and factually.

To reduce the level of anxiety and help her become more comfortable.	3) Anxious, fearful and preoccupied:
	a) Talks rapidly in a loud tone of voice.
	b) Repeats herself.
	c) Asks nurses to repeat says, "I didn't hear."
		5) Speak
		  a) Clearly
		  b) Slowly
		  c) Briefly
		  d) In a quiet tone
		6) Ask for and answer questions in a friendly, unhurried manner.
			Anxiety occurs when one is confronted with a situation which threatens one's self-image.	

290

TABLE 21-1 (continued)

NAME: Sheila Franklin NURSE: Miss Maris DATE: 3/1/19___

Nursing Care Goals	Patient Problems	Nursing Intervention	Rationale	Results of Intervention
	d) Possible refusal of h.s. medication because she is afraid to sleep with door unlocked.	7) Has Beta-chlor capsule ordered for h.s.: a) Withhold h.s. medication until night nurse is on duty. b) Introduce night nurse. c) Have night nurse (Miss Jeffrey) explain: 1) Night rounds 2) Cleaning details 3) Possible unexpected sounds	A moderate degree of anxiety produces a decrease in perception. Therefore, clear, brief, repeated communications are needed to lessen level of anxiety and increase sense of trust.	Accepted the sedatives after being reassured that rounds were really made.

morning report: 3/2/19___

Miss Jeffrey, the night nurse, reported that Mrs. Franklin had agreed to take the sedative ordered after being assured that the door to her room could be kept closed. Mrs. Franklin was awake twice during the night. The first time was at 2 a.m.; as the nurse entered the room, Mrs. Franklin said, "I'm still awake." But before the nurse could respond Mrs. Franklin was already asleep again. The second time occurred about 4:30 a.m. This time when the nurse entered her room, Mrs. Franklin wanted to know if it was time to get up.

Miss Jeffrey related that Miss Valor, the evening nurse assigned to Mrs. Franklin, had reported that Mrs. Franklin had refused to go to the lounge but that she did agree to meet Mrs. Jones, a patient in the room next to hers and that Mrs. Franklin stayed to talk with Mrs. Jones for a few minutes. Miss Valor spent about a half an hour talking with Mrs. Franklin and learned that she liked to read—romantic, adventure and historical novels. She also discovered that Mrs. Franklin did some painting when she was in school but had not had much time for it since her little girl was born. She does sew for herself and Debby: "simple things—nothing too complicated."

After the scheduled ward team conference, Miss Maris and the head nurse conducted the nursing care conference to spell out the nursing care goals, identify the problems and plan specific nursing interventions. The nursing care plan they developed (Table 21-2) reflects the philosophy and treatment plan of the entire ward team.

TABLE 21-2
NURSING CARE PLAN II

NAME: Sheila Franklin NURSE: Miss Maris DATE: 3/2/19

Nursing Care Goals	Patient Problems	Nursing Intervention	Rationale	Results of Intervention
To create and maintain an environment which reflects an attitude of honesty, support and genuine concern for patient needs. To increase feelings of security through a climate which demonstrates acceptance of the individual.	1) Suspiciousness	1) Show acceptance by being: a) Scrupulously honest. 1) Respond with correct, accurate information to questions. 2) Explain routines and procedures clearly. 3) Keep promises. b) Consistent, friendly and persistent. 1) Initiate approaches. 2) Assign particular staff members: a) Days—Miss Maris, R.N. b) Evenings—Miss Valor, R.N. c) Nights—Miss Jeffrey, R.N.	Attitudes and actions indicating that an individual is worthy of attention or concern contribute to a feeling of being cared about.	

TABLE 21-2 (continued)

NAME: Sheila Franklin   NURSE: Miss Maris   DATE: 3/2/19___

Nursing Care Goals	Patient Problems	Nursing Intervention	Rationale	Results of Intervention
To provide reality orientation for patient.	2) Withdrawn	2) Plan schedule with patient and adhere to it: a) Rising—7:30 a.m. 　1) Wash and dress before breakfast. 　2) Give positive recognition when Mrs. F. complies with policy regarding clothes. b) Bath—10 p.m. Prefers tub bath 3) Meals a) Inform about dining hours: 7:30-9:00; 11:30-1:00; 4:30-6:00 b) Observe eating habits; amount, selection, and frequency.	Familiar routines and persons contribute to a sense of security. Commitment to a schedule is a base for developing a successful identity, and decreases the fear of the unknown thereby promoting security. Modification of hospital routines assist in individualizing care and demonstrates to the patient the staff's concern.	Skips lunch

294

TABLE 21-2 (continued)

NAME: Sheila Franklin NURSE: Miss Maris DATE: 3/2/19___

Nursing Care Goals	Patient Problems	Nursing Intervention	Rationale	Results of Intervention
		c) Encourage to sit with Mrs. Jones in dining room. (Be sure chair faces door.)		Agreed to sit at the same table with Mrs. Jones. Responds but does not initiate conversation.
		d) Evening snack—8:30 p.m.		
		4) Medications		
		a) Thorazine 100 mgm. b.i.d. 9 a.m.–9 p.m.		
		b) Beta-Chlor Capsule at 11 p.m. prn		
		1) Observe and record response to medications.		
		2) Discuss medication with Mrs. F.		
To identify, explore and demonstrate to the individual satisfactory and effective ways of establishing and maintaining interpersonal relationships.		5) Counseling session: 1:00–1:30 daily with Miss Maris.	Limitation of number of staff contacts is important because ability of patient to trust is lacking.	
		6) Occupational Therapy: 10–11:30 daily	Collaboration with other disciplines provides for consistency and continuity of care.	Looking at blouse patterns, Mrs. F. said she might make herself a blouse. Therapist re-
		a) Miss Maris to escort and introduce patient first time.		

TABLE 21-2 (continued)

NAME: Sheila Franklin NURSE: Miss Maris DATE: 3/2/19___

Nursing Care Goals	Patient Problems	Nursing Intervention	Rationale	Results of Intervention
		b) Supply therapist with additional needed information.		ported that patient sat and looked at patterns but couldn't make a decision.
		c) Confer with therapist on regular basis for a mutual exchange regarding progress.		
To provide continuing support, reassurance and teaching to the patient and his family.		7) Visitors—2–4; 7–9 daily:		
		a) Observe interaction between patient and visitors.		
		b) Talk with visitors and acquaint them with regulations of ward.		
		c) Answer questions for visitors.		
		8) Recreational Therapy: 7–8:30 on ward		
		9) Rest periods or Free Time: 1:30–2:00 p.m. 4:00–4:30 p.m. 6:30–7:00 and 9–10 p.m.		

TABLE 21-2 (continued)

NAME: Sheila Franklin   NURSE: Miss Maris   DATE: 3/2/19____

Nursing Care Goals	Patient Problems	Nursing Intervention	Rationale	Results of Intervention

To help develop within the patient a realistic and positive self concept from which healthy feelings of self-esteem and self-respect would emerge.	3) Patient remains secluded.	10) Retiring—after the 11 p.m. news
		
		11) Approach and invite Mrs. F. to leave her room during free periods.
		  a) Stay with her for a few minutes each time she refuses.
		  b) Recognize it may take time before she is willing to leave her room.
		  c) Try positive suggestions:
		    1) I'd like, ____
		    2) I need, ____
		    3) I'd appreciate
			To experience satisfying relationships with others, the individual must be able to feel that he will not be harmed by the relationship.	Says she stays in her room because she needs quiet to read. However she is unable to discuss her book.

To help the patient to experss feelings of hostility constructively and in a safe acceptable manner.	4) Hostility: Responds in an abrupt, critical and sarcastic manner to head nurse, nursing assistants and physician.	12) Become aware of, anticipate and observe negative feelings and behavior. a) Observe for signs of mounting hostility:	Hostility is usually a negative response which occurs when one's sense of independence is threatened, particularly in relationships with authority figures.	

297

TABLE 21-2 (continued)

NAME: Sheila Franklin NURSE: Miss Maris DATE: 3/2/19___

Nursing Care Goals	Patient Problems	Nursing Intervention	Rationale	Results of Intervention
		1) Listen to complaints without making excuses or becoming angry. 2) Keep calm. b) Help Mrs. F. to identify specific cues to hostility: 1) Allow and encourage Mrs. F. to discuss the situation: a) What happened and when did it occur? b. What provoked the behavior? c. Who was involved? 2) How did Mrs. F. express her feelings? 3) What might she do next time?	Discussion of hostility producing situations allows the individual to identify feelings and behavior without fear of judgment or retaliation. It also provides an opportunity for learning alternate methods of responding which will increase feelings of satisfaction.	

evaluation of care

On March 8th, at the end of the first week of hospitalization, the nursing care plan was reviewed, evaluated and revised. Mrs. Franklin is not completely adhering to the planned schedule. She goes to the dining room for breakfast and dinner; skips lunch and refuses the evening snack. She usually wakes up once during the night. The first two days Mrs. Franklin received Thorazine she complained of feeling sleepy and noted some dryness of the mouth. Mrs. Franklin attends occupational therapy but is still looking at the pattern book and is unable to decide what she is going to make. The recreational therapy sessions in the evenings were refused with such excuses as: "I would rather read; I cannot dance; I do not like to play games." Mrs. Franklin is not as abrupt with the nursing staff but she did tell at least two patients who approached her and asked her to join them in a card game, to "mind their own business." The staff agreed to give priority to:

I) focusing the nurse-patient interaction on:
  1) Mrs. Franklin's inability to relate with other people as evidenced by her non-involvement in ward activities and,
  2) identifying those factors which seem to prevent Mrs. Franklin from assuming the necessary responsibility for committing herself to decision-making.

II) introducing those solitary activities which have been identified as successful experiences in the past.

Mrs. Franklin was asked to join the nursing staff conference to discuss these treatment goals and the way in which they could be implemented with her. The following revision of the nursing care plan was developed and a time was set for evaluation of progress. (Table 21-3)

TABLE 21-3
NURSING CARE PLAN III

NAME: Sheila Franklin NURSE: Miss Maris DATE: 3/9/19___

Nursing Care Goals	Patient Problems	Nursing Intervention	Rationale	Results of Intervention
To allow Mrs. Franklin to verbalize and examine her inability to become involved in activity.	1) Nonparticipation	1) Continue daily nurse-patient interaction. a) Increase time to one hour. b) Try two half sessions: one in the morning, and one in afternoon. 2) Approach patient at the beginning of each scheduled activity. a) Talk with her about the situation. b) Encourage participation by joining her in the activity.	Demonstration of continued acceptance toward patient results in lessening of suspicion and provides opportunities for testing reality.	Kept two morning sessions, but made excuses for avoiding the afternoon sessions. Would agree to participate; start an activity, but lose interest after 15-20 minutes.
To experience success, reinforce self-esteem and prevent regression.	2) Hostility toward other patients. 3) Excessive use of rationalization. 4) Misinterprets motives of others.	3) Provide meaningful tasks and assistance in: a) Occupational Therapy: 1) Selecting a pattern 2) Arranging for buying fabric	Identifying achievements and positively acknowledging her accomplishments will foster feelings of adequacy and increase her self-confidence.	Selected two patterns and agreed to go to shopping center with nurse.

TABLE 21-3 (continued)

NAME: Sheila Franklin   NURSE: Miss Maris   DATE: 3/9/19 _____

Nursing Care Goals	Patient Problems	Nursing Intervention	Rationale	Results of Intervention
		3) Pinning and cutting the fabric 4) Completing the task. b) On the ward: 1) To maintain typing skills obtain a type writer for her to use. 2) Request that Mrs. F. type ward lists, bed charts, time sheets, etc.	Providing an opportunity to demonstrate real skills and earn appropriate recognition.	Complained she can't type lists because of staff's illegible writing. Became angry when Miss Maris offered to read lists to her and said, "You're just like my boss, setting impossible tasks."
		3) Ask for her assistance in maintaining the ward library: a) Arrange books on shelf b) Dispose of outdated magazines and newspapers c) Buy daily newspaper in hospital lobby.		Arranged all books upside down. Threw out *all* magazines.

a crisis situation

On March 12th at 3:20 a.m., Mrs. Jeffrey heard a scream coming from the direction of Mrs. Franklin's room. On investigation, the nurse found Mrs. Franklin cowering in her bed. As Mrs. Jeffrey approached Mrs. Franklin, she could hear her whimpering over and over, "No! No! Stay away from me! You're dead! Dead!" Mrs. Franklin sobbed and mumbled incoherently for approximately fifteen minutes. When asked what was happening, Mrs. Franklin denied that anything was the matter. As the nurse tried to focus on the incident and her outcry, Mrs. Franklin insisted that she was all right saying, "It's nothing, just a nightmare! I'm fine." Miss Jeffrey got Mrs. Franklin a glass of warm milk and sat with her until she dropped off to sleep again. The nurse checked on her every half hour and found that Mrs. Franklin was sleeping but was restless. When Mrs. Jeffrey entered Mrs. Franklin's room at 5:30 a.m., she found her lying rigidly, staring up at the ceiling and nonresponsive to verbal communication.

The nursing staff held a short conference to plan for immediate revision of the nursing care plan and goals previously set for Mrs. Franklin's care. The changes were based on Mrs. Jeffrey's report and the observations Miss Maris made during her morning rounds. During the conference, the goals were revised and the nursing staff discussed their own feeling and reactions to Mrs. Franklin's apparent setback. The priorities they established at this time were identifed as:

1 Limit the regression by encouraging Mrs. Franklin to focus outside self.
2 Meet dependency needs while encouraging and assisting in activities of daily living.
3 Convey the expectation of resuming full functioning in a short period of time.
4 Encourage her to verbalize her feelings.

A revised nursing care plan (Table 21-4) was initiated for Mrs. Franklin.

TABLE 21-4
NURSING CARE PLAN IV

NAME: Sheila Franklin NURSE: Miss Maris DATE: 3/12/19__

Nursing Care Goals	Patient Problems	Nursing Intervention	Rationale	Results of Intervention
To limit regression and focus on reality orientation.	1) Immobile. 2) Body rigid. 3) Staring at ceiling. 4) Mute.	1) Assign counseling nurse to provide total care. (Miss Maris) a) Approach in a matter-of-fact manner. b) Be patient and understanding. c) Demonstrate concern: "Mrs. Franklin, something happened last night. Perhaps you'll tell me . . ." 1) Sit quietly. 2) Allow ample time for the patient to respond. 3) "I'll spend more time with you today. Maybe later . . ." 4) "Now, I'll help you get ready for breakfast."	Regression is a means of relieving anxiety. Collapse of adult behavioral patterns occurs as frustration and conflict increases. Concerted effort in terms of staff attitude are required to influence the degree and time span of the regressive process. Direct verbal communications are used to focus on reality.	Followed movements of nurse with eyes but did not move head.

303

TABLE 21-4 (continued)

NAME: Sheila Franklin   NURSE: Miss Maris   DATE: 3/12/19___

Nursing Care Goals	Patient Problems	Nursing Intervention	Rationale	Results of Intervention

To meet dependency needs and make reality more comfortable.		2) Make no demands this morning.
		a) Give positive instructions:
		  1) Personal hygiene:
		    a) "Wash and dry your face and hands."
		    b) "It's time to brush your teeth."
		    c) "Comb your hair."
		  2) Breakfast—Lunch:
		    a) "Drink your juice, Mrs. F."
		    b) "Eat the oatmeal."
		    c) "Shall I add cream and sugar to your coffee?"
		  b) Prepare any articles needed for use such as wash cloth, towels, tooth brush, meal tray, and eating utensils.
			Expression of intense dependence connotes a need for recognition and attention.
			
			Equilibrium is restored when dependency needs are met.
				Took fifteen minutes to wash face and hands. No verbal response.
				
				Drank juice, ate half serving of oatmeal, refused toast and eggs. Nodded head negatively. Refused lunch.

TABLE 21-4 (continued)

NAME: Sheila Franklin   NURSE: Miss Maris   DATE: 3/12/19

Nursing Care Goals	Patient Problems	Nursing Intervention	Rationale	Results of Intervention
		c) Offer assistance if unable to do for self: 1) Bathe, comb hair, apply make-up. 2) Prepare meal tray. 3) Feed.		
		d) Offer and encourage fruit juices several times during the day.	To prevent the possibility of dehydration.	Total fluid intake from 7:30 a.m. to 1:00 p.m. was 500 cc.
To help her maintain her feelings of personal worth.		3) Approach Mrs. Franklin every hour for at least fifteen minutes each time during remainder of the day. a) Address her by name. b) Mention the time limits: "Mrs. F. it's 10 a.m. I'll be here for fifteen minutes. I'll sit and talk with you now." c) Wait for response: 1) Sit quietly in silence.	Continuous interest, persistence and "there-ness" of the nurse communicates a concern and willingness to help.	Nonresponsive on verbal level. No eye contact.

TABLE 21-4 (continued)

NAME: Sheila Franklin   NURSE: Miss Maris   DATE: 3/12/19___

Nursing Care Goals	Patient Problems	Nursing Intervention	Rationale	Results of Intervention

		2) Focus attention on patient.
		3) Make short, nonanxiety producing statements.
		  a) "I'll be in and out to see you throughout the morning."
		  b) "I'll bring a magazine for us to look at next time."
		  c) "I'll be here five more minutes."
				Became rigid when approached with own clothes. Allowed self to be dressed in bathrobe; was helped out of bed.

To gradually increase activity and responsibility.		4) Encourage and assist Mrs. Franklin to get dressed in the afternoon. 5) Provide solitary activities: a) Furnish two or three current magazines focusing on previous expressed interests:	Simple, solitary activities reduce stress and promote comfort.	

TABLE 21-4 (continued)

NAME: Sheila Franklin NURSE: Miss Maris DATE: 3/12/19___

Nursing Care Goals	Patient Problems	Nursing Intervention	Rationale	Results of Intervention
		1) *Vogue* 2) *Ladies Home Journal* 3) *Good Housekeeping*		
		b) Page through the magazine and attempt to elicit Mrs. Franklin's comments on color, styles, recipes, etc.	Activities are an effective means of encouraging self-expression.	Would not turn pages or look at magazine.
		c) Secure finger paints from O.T. and introduce to Mrs. F.		Smeared finger paints over self and clothes. Permitted nurse to wash hands and face. Threw puzzle on floor. Refused to leave room.
		d) Set up a small colorful picture puzzle of no more than 25-30 pieces.	Increasing responsibility implies a therapeutic optimism and expectation of patient participation in routine.	
		e) Offer to accompany Mrs. F. on a short walk in the hallway.		

progress report

Mrs. Franklin remained mute and demanded a great deal of assistance in meeting her most basic, elementary needs. Bathing and dressing was a very slow process which required detailed instructions, encouragement and supervision from the nurse every step of the way. Reminders to eat, to take her medications and to go to the bathroom were constantly reiterated.

The physician decided to increase Mrs. Franklin's medication and the Thorazine order was changed to 100 mg. Q.I.D. Miss Maris observed that Mrs. Franklin noted the change in medication as evidenced by her questioning glance at the nurse when she brought them to her at 1:00 and 5:00 in the afternoon. Mrs. Franklin did not make any comment when Miss Maris pointed out the change.

Since Mrs. Franklin still had not spoken after three days, the staff decided that Miss Maris should provide her with a notebook and suggest to her that she write in diary form her thoughts and feelings. Miss Maris tried to convey the attitude that she understood how difficult it was to talk about some things. She told Mrs. Franklin that it might even be painful. However, sometimes writing one's thoughts and feelings might make it easier to share them. Miss Maris offered to help her identify those thoughts and feelings which might be causing her present discomfort. The nurse also suggested that together they could explore these concerns and work out possible solutions.

Because of the intensive demonstration of concern displayed by the entire staff, the regressive period was interrupted after five days. Gradually, Mrs. Franklin was able to resume functioning at a level comparable to that which existed prior to the crisis situation.

From this point on the staff, Mrs. Franklin and her family were actively involved in trying out different methods to deal more effectively with her fears, feelings of guilt and suspiciousness. The plan provided for gradual resocialization through increasing Mrs. Franklin's contact with selected patients and other staff members both on and off the ward. Initially, competition was avoided or kept to a minimum. As the patient developed more self-confidence, she was included in daily group therapy sessions to further provide positive feedback in developing relationships with others.

therapeutic communication:
a nurse-patient interaction with mrs. franklin

An actual nurse-patient interaction between Miss Maris and Mrs. Franklin is reported here (Table 21-5) to provide an example of an effective therapeutic nurse-patient communication process. Inclusion of this sample will demonstrate:

1 The use of a therapeutic relationship as means of carrying out the nursing care goals.

2 The use of a counseling session as part of the total treatment process.

3 How the techniques of communication can be used effectively in the practical application of a theoretical framework.

4 The way in which the nurse and patient together identify a problem area and seek a workable solution.

5 The way in which the learning process is implemented to bring about a desired change in behavior.

6 The part evaluation plays in determining effective communication.

7 The planning for subsequent sessions based on achievements of mutually derived goals.

TABLE 21-5
NURSE-PATIENT INTERACTION

| Patient Name | Mrs. Sheila Franklin | Date 3/20/19___ |
| Nurse Name | Miss Maris | Number of Interactions 35th Hour |

GOALS:

1) For Patient:
a) Continue to explore and describe manifestations of her anxiety and anger.
b) Recognize the precipitating factors in the development of her anxiety.
c) Identify one or more ways to cope with the expressed feelings.

2) For Nurse:
a) Use therapeutic techniques appropriately.
b) Allow Mrs. Franklin as much time as she needs to think and respond.
c) Identify my own thoughts, feelings and behavior as Mrs. Franklin talks about stressful situations with which I am familiar.

Nurse	Patient	Comments	Evaluation
"Good Morning Mrs. F."	"Good Morning. I'm ready. Where do we begin today?"	Give recognition. Mrs. F. was eager to begin today's session. Looked bright. Greeted me with a half smile.	I did not respond to question. Allowed Mrs. Franklin time to assume the initiative.
"You sound pleased."	"I've actually gained five pounds since last week. I think I've gained this much because I'm eating better. My appetite is enormous. I even eat lunch now I am, but—oh well, it doesn't matter."	Translating into feelings. First time Mrs. F. has spoken of her weight. Signs of positive feelings about self. Grimaces, shrugs shoulders and looks disgusted.	

TABLE 21-5 (continued)

Nurse	Patient	Comments	Evaluation
"What doesn't matter?"	"If I continue to gain weight I won't have any clothes to wear. I don't have a job. I can't afford to buy new clothes. I can't depend on my parents forever. My insurance money is almost all gone."	Exploring. Expresses concern over welfare. Sounds distressed.	
"You're really worried about this?"	"Well, wouldn't you be? What do you do when you don't have any money? It's important to have money, without it, how can I care for Debby?"	Verbalize the implied. Mrs. F. avoided a direct response and focused on the nurse. Gives second reason for needing money. May feel threatened by possibility of returning to work.	
"What do you think you could do?"	"Go to work, I guess, How can I go to work or even look for a job. I'm stuck in this place."	Reflecting. Tone of voice is harsh and angry.	Allow her to pursue these factors and focus on threat later.
"You seem to have two areas of concern, getting a job and leaving the hospital. Let's talk about the job first."	(Mrs. F. nods head affirmatively)	Patient quiet. I waited about two minutes before continuing. Verbalizing the implied and asking for clarification.	

TABLE 21-5 (continued)

Nurse	Patient	Comments	Evaluation
"You've worked as a secretary before."	"Yes, but not for the last year or so. I used to be a pretty good typist and I could do shorthand but I can't concentrate anymore."	Focusing and setting priority. Asking her to collaborate with me to pursue one problem at a time. Offering a broad opening, or general lead from nurse's knowledge of patient's background. Some basis in fact for feelings of inadequacy, however has helped with ward typing and does job well. Some elements of rationalization. Increased level of anxiety noted or evidenced by restless movements in chair, play with buttons on blouse and looking out window.	
"Can't concentrate or feel uncomfortable because you're out of practice? You sound angry . . ."	"It doesn't matter, does it? I'm stuck in this hospital."	Seeking clarification. Picked up nonverbal cues of discomfort. Looks angry. Sounds sarcastic.	Did not help Mrs. F. to recognize increasing anxiety. Discomfort continues to increase resulting in angry outburst.
	I'm better now than I've ever been before. I know it. I feel it.	Verbalizing implied feelings. Leans forward in chair. Looks directly at nurse. Statement said with conviction and firmness.	
	. . . But I wonder if I can handle a job. I've been away so long."	Reflects feelings of inadequacy.	Possible demonstration of ambivalence.

TABLE 21-5 (continued)

Nurse	Patient	Comments	Evaluation
You're afraid—"	"Yes, I'm afraid. I know that I'm strong enough physically and mentally. I worry, I'm nervous and I used to get upset at work before. You know, working in an office with a bunch of other girls isn't conducive to good nerves. I've had people tell me—'Boy, I wouldn't have your job for anything.' But, you work with a lot of women too. Don't you run into the same kind of problems?"	Translating her thoughts into feelings. Able to recognize and name the anxiety. This is the first step in the learning process.	The next step in the learning process would be to encourage her to describe her feelings of "nervousness."
		Use of rationalization.	
		Giggled. Evidence again of increased discomfort.	
		Tries to decrease feelings of uncomfortableness by shifting focus onto the nurse.	
		Indirectly asking for agreement rather than looking at self in relation to situation.	
"What kind of problem?"	"Oh! You know! Someone expecting you to do more than the next guy. In my last job, I didn't mind helping out once in awhile, staying over and doing the last minute jobs. But a couple of the girls were young and had boy friends, they had dates or plans so most of the time they wouldn't stay. The other lady was married and had small children so she had a good excuse for leaving on	Exploration.	I avoided being trapped into agreement.
		Automatic knowing is a part of magical thinking. This account of behavior and expectations of her co-workers toward her fed into her feelings of suspiciousness and could be the basis for some of her delusions of persecution and ideas of reference.	

TABLE 21-5 (continued)

Nurse	Patient	Comments	Evaluation
	time. That left me to work all the extra, 'cause they figured I'm a widow. Mom is there to look after Debby so I didn't have a good excuse."		Tried to remain objective.
"Did this happen often?"	"Often enough. I kept track the last month I worked, it happened five times out of two weeks."	Placing events in sequence.	This technique was used in order to begin to help her make comparisons.
"Do you recall what you were feeling when each of these situations occurred?"	"Overworked, tired, mad! I remember one time especially. I was really feeling bad; my head hurt, I was sneezing and my eyes burned I thought I was catching a cold. The boss wanted three letters typed and mailed before morning. They all said, 'Sheila will do them.' I felt rotten but I got the letters out."	Asking for description of feelings. Limited ability to describe. Uses broad, general terms. Mrs. F. has a pattern of handling anxiety through the development of physical symptoms. She uses illness as a rationalization to explain her behavior.	Asked for a description of feelings to help her complete the second step of the learning process.
"Then what happened?"	"Then I went home and went to bed. I didn't even eat supper. I slept through 'til 10	Offering a general lead to encourage her to continue. Extreme fatigue without feeling rested connotes high level of anxiety.	

TABLE 21-5 (continued)

Nurse	Patient	Comments	Evaluation
	o'clock the next morning but I didn't care. I didn't go to work until noon that day."	Behavior demonstrates withdrawal as a coping mechanism.	
"You seem very uncomfortable about the situation you just described."		Manifests anxiety in retrospect.	Tried to get Mrs. F. to take a look at the way she deals with situations which produce anger.
"Earlier in today's session you said, 'I'm better now than I've ever been before'."	"Yes, that's right! And I still think so! Before when this happened I got sick and mad. I mean really mad!"	Making observation and encouraging comparison and evaluation. Emphatic.	Realizes differences in degree of felt anger. Recognizes the influence of her feelings on her behavior. This awareness demonstrates increasing amounts of insight.
"And now?"	"Now, I guess I'll say I get upset when I think about people using me. Before I couldn't do anything different but be mad. Now, I do get mad but its different."	Encouraging evaluation. Pauses, looking angry. Appears thoughtful. Expression changes to one of determination. Making comparisons and noting differences, which is the third step in the learning process.	Nurse feels like she could take a bow. Overjoyed with the patient's progress.
"Different—in what way?"	"I used to feel tied up in knots when I was angry. I'd shut	Encouraging comparison and asking for further de-	

TABLE 21-5 (continued)

Nurse	Patient	Comments	Evaluation
	myself away in my room. I'd feel sick and go to bed. I still feel tight but its not so bad. Like the other day when Mrs. Jones came in and picked up my diary. I got mad. I felt like I wanted to push her out. Instead I said, 'That's a very personal thing and I prefer you don't look at it.' She apologized and put it down. Then we started talking about something else."	scription of perceptions. Able to supply a specific example to illustrate comparison.	Patient's use of an alternative acceptable method of dealing with anger met with success.
"You feel this is different?"	"Oh yes! I told somebody what I really thought and it worked out okay. I didn't get sick."	Mrs. F. sounded surprised. Encouraging evaluation. Stated with confidence.	Patient has recognized that she has learned a new method of coping.
"That really is different."	"It sure is—I feel that I can do something about it now."	Presenting reality. Sounds pleased with self. Acknowledges difference. Continues after slight pause.	
"Like what?"	"Well, I don't have to let people use me."	Exploring. To help Mrs. F. formulate a plan of action for dealing with her discomfort and anger.	

TABLE 21-5 (continued)

Nurse	Patient	Comments	Evaluation
"Go on."		General lead.	
	"If I don't feel like doing something I could say no or tell them I don't like what they are doing."	Hesitated briefly before responding then let the words rush out.	
"How do you feel about saying no?"		Encouraging description of perception.	
	"I never thought about it, I guess. I've never liked to say no but I found out it doesn't hurt."	Perplexed. Conveys a sense of insecurity but a willingness to try.	Needs continued support and reassurance. Possibly plan opportunities where she can further test out her solution. May need help with developing compromises in some situations.
"How would you apply this to the work situation you described earlier?"		Encouraging comparison and evaluation. Helping Mrs. F. to formulate a plan of action.	
	"I guess now I would feel more confident. I could take a chance and say no when I don't want to work over."	Sounds more sure of self and action to be taken.	
"What would you do if your co-workers did not go along with your no?"		Presenting reality.	
	"Well, I don't know—I'll have to think about that—"	Realistic approach to unknown situation. Decision demonstrates ability to plan	

317

TABLE 21-5 (continued)

Nurse	Patient	Comments	Evaluation
"Perhaps next time we could explore this point further."		action rather than respond impulsively. Encourage formulation of a plan of action. Setting up goal for next interaction session.	
"Mrs. Franklin, there's five minutes remaining in the session. As you and I talked, it became evident that you had two important areas of concern, getting a job and your continued hospitalization. In the course of our discussion you identified your feelings of nervousness and anger on the job. You explored these in detail and gave me the impression that you can better deal with these feelings now. I am pleased to hear this."		Summarizing. Organizing the important points of the interaction.	
	"I feel pretty proud of myself too."		
"On Wednesday we can discuss your getting a job and feelings about leaving the hospital."		Giving recognition, acknowledgment and merited praise to Mrs. Franklin's accomplishment of a difficult task.	
	"See you Wednesday."		

evaluation of interaction by miss maris

"As I reviewed this interaction immediately after the session, I was convinced that the total interaction clearly demonstrates that we are in the working phase of the therapeutic relationship. Mrs. Franklin's responses indicated that she felt secure and was able to verbalize her real feelings. This made me feel very good. I felt I had accomplished a major task. The areas which require additional work on my part to make the process more therapeutic are:

1 using more reflection in order to elicit and clarify her feelings,
2 allowing Mrs. Franklin more time to express her feeling before I attempt to translate her comments into feelings, and
3 to broaden my use of a variety of therapeutic techniques of communication.

With respect to Mrs. Franklin I think that she needs:

1 exposure to a variety of situations where she can experiment with testing her reactions and responses,
2 reinforcement of the learning process as a means of dealing effectively with uncomfortable situations and
3 time to deliberate and validate her feelings with others.

Mrs. Franklin shows an increased ability to deal more effectively with current living situations. She displays an interest in self, concern for her appearance, an awareness of financial responsibility all of which indicates to me an increase in her level of independence. She is also showing signs of irritability concerning continued hospitalization which seems to me to be a readiness to move constructively toward discharge. In the next two sessions, I will prepare for her inclusion into the family counseling sessions I am presently having with her parents and brother."

summary report

After an additional two weeks in group therapy, Mrs. Franklin was included in the family counseling sessions with her parents and brother. She met with Miss Maris and her family a total of four times over the next two weeks. As a result of these meetings, Mrs. Franklin was able to scan the want ads and initiate calls to placement agencies for job interviews. The brother supported Mrs. Franklin by agreeing to provide transportation to the interviews. She joined a Parents Without Partners group which is active in her community. She attended her first meeting while still hospitalized and requested that Miss Maris accompany her. The school counselor was contacted because the grandparents expressed concern that Debby "is not doing her work, she is afraid to go to bed at night and she cries a lot."

At the end of Mrs. Franklin's seventh week of hospitalization, the ward team met to finalize discharge plans with her. Mrs. Franklin was discharged one week later. Arrangements were made through referral for her to attend weekly group therapy sessions in a nearby mental health clinic. Miss Maris was to maintain contact and to visit in the home once a month until such time as Mrs. Franklin would be able to function more independently and complete the termination phase of the nurse-patient relationship.

Approximately nine months after hospitalization, Miss Maris discontinued the home visits and reassured Mrs. Franklin that she could keep in touch via the telephone. Mrs. Franklin is working as a secretary and is now dating a widower with two children.

suggested readings

Beyers, Virginia B. *Nursing Observation.* Wm. C. Brown Co.: Dubuque, Iowa, 1970.

Carlson, Sylvia. "A Practical Approach to the Nursing Process." *American Journal of Nursing,* Vol. 72 No. 9 (September, 1972), 1589-1591.

Carter, Joan Haselman, et al. *Standards of Nursing Care: A Guide to Evaluation.* Springer Publishing Co., Inc.: New York 1972.

Davidson, Jean M. "Concept and Utilization of Multimedia Laboratory in a Community Registered Nursing Program." *The Journal of Nursing Education,* Vol. 72 No. 1 (January, 1972).

Eggland, Ellen Thomas. "How to Take a Meaningful History." *Nursing '77,* Vol. 7 No. 7 (July, 1977), 22-30.

Eisenman, Elaine, Backer, Barbara A., and Dubbert, Patricia M. "The Mental Health Assessment Interview." *Psychiatric/Mental Health Nursing: Contemporary Readings.* D. Van Nostrand Company, Inc.: New York, 1978, 7-30.

————. "Gaining Insight Into Fear." *Nursing '78,* Vol. 8 No. 4 (April, 1978), 46-51.

Geach, Barbara. "The Problem-Solving Technique as Taught to Psychiatric Nursing Students." *Perspectives in Psychiatric Care,* Vol. 12 No. 1 (January/March, 1974), 9-12.

King, Joan M. "The Initial Interview—Assessment of the Patient and His Difficulties." *Perspectives in Psychiatric Care.* Vol. 5 No. 6 (1967), 256-261.

Little, Dolores E., and Carnevoli, Doria L. *Nursing Care Planning.* J. B. Lippincott Co.: Philadelphia, 1969.

Manfreda, Marquerite L. *Psychiatric Nursing.* 9th ed. F. A. Davis Co.: Philadelphia, 1977.

Mayers, Marlene G. *A Systematic Approach to the Nursing Care Plan.* Appleton-Century-Crofts: Meredith Corporation, 1972.

Miller, Sister Patricia. "Clinical Knowledge: A Needed Curriculum Emphasis." *Nursing Outlook,* Vol. 23 No. 4 (April, 1975).

McCain, R. Faye. "Nursing by Assessment—Not Intuition." *American Journal of Nursing,* Vol. 65 No. 4 (April, 1965), 82-84.

McClosky, Joanne C. "How to Make The Most of Body Image Theory in Nursing Practice." *Nursing '76,* Vol. 6, 68-72.

Murray, Ruth, and Zintner, Judith. *Nursing Assessment and Health Promotion Through the Life Span.* Prentice-Hall, Inc.: Englewood Cliffs, New Jersey, 1975.

Nursing Action Guide. Committee on Research in Clinical Nursing, U.S. Government Printing Office, Washington, D.C., 1970.

Schwartz, Morris S., and Shockley, Emmy L. *The Nurse and the Mental Patient.* John Wiley and Sons: New York, 1956.

Sloboda, Sharon. "Understanding Patient Behavior." *Nursing '77,* Vol. 7 No. 9 (September, 1977), 74-77.

Snyder, Cameron Joyce, and Wilson, Foltz Margo. "Elements of a Psychological Assessment." *American Journal of Nursing,* Vol. 77 No. 2 (February, 1977), 235-239.

Standards: Psychiatric-Mental Health Nursing Practice. American Nurses Association, Kansas City, Missouri, 1973.

Trail, Ira Davis. *Establishing Relationships in Psychiatric Nursing.* Springer Publishing Co., Inc.: New York, 1966.

Turnbull, Sister Joyce. "Shifting The Focus To Health." *American Journal of Nursing,* Vol. 76 No. 12 (December, 1976), 1985-1987.

glossary

Acting out The behavioral expression of fantasies, feelings or conflicts through unconventional actions.

Addiction Strong uncontrolled psychophysiological dependence on the effects of substances which when taken into the body provide temporary relief from emotional discomfort.

Advocacy An attitude of support to protect the integrity and safeguard the rights of the patient.

Affect A generalized, persistent and pervasive feeling tone.

Aggression Destructive goal-directed behavior closely associated with anger.

Ambivalence The simultaneous existence of contrary emotions, values, attitudes or desires toward an object or person.

Anxiety A feeling state in which the individual experiences pervasive, vague, intense sensations of apprehension of impending disaster.

Apathy A state of indifference or absence of affective response.

Assessment A process whereby the nurse gathers and examines all data pertinent to the patient and his illness.

Attitude An opinion or viewpoint with which a person consistently and persistently confronts other persons and related situations.

Autism The complete exclusion of reality through preoccupation and absorption in fantasy within the self.

Behavior A set of actions characteristic to an individual which can be observed and recorded.

Blocking A sudden interruption in the stream of thought.

Body language Nonverbal communication in which the individual expresses his thoughts, feelings and attitudes through the use of physical means such as facial expressions, gestures, posture, movement, tone of voice or touch.

Communication A social process involving an interchange of ideas between two or more people.

Compulsion The uncontrollable urge to perform repetitive acts despite one's better judgment.

Confabulation The invention and recounting of plausible explanations to conceal memory gaps.

Conflict A feeling state, either conscious or unconscious, in which the individual experiences a clash between two or more equally strong, opposing forces.

Conscious That part of the mind or state of awareness which is necessary for adapting to and making use of one's environment.

Coping The ability to adapt and adjust to changing life situations.

Crisis A situation or a problem with which the individual is not able to cope through usual or ordinary means.

Crisis intervention Short term treatment directed toward assisting the individual to solve his immediate problems.

Delusion A fixed false belief which cannot be corrected through logical reasoning. Four common types include:

Delusion of grandeur A fixed false belief in which the patient portrays an exaggerated feeling of importance in terms of wealth, power or influence.

Delusion of persecution A fixed false belief in which the patient claims that others are against him or are about to harm him.

Somatic delusions A fixed false belief in which the patient maintains that his body is disturbed or disordered in one or all of its parts.

Delusions of reference A fixed false belief in which the patient avows that the words or actions of others have special meaning and are specifically directed toward him.

Depersonalization A denying of one's own personal identity; a feeling of being different, strange or unreal.

Depression An intense pervasive feeling of sadness or dejection.

Disorientation An impaired recognition and understanding of temporal, spatial or personal relationships.

Dissociation Cutting off or compartmentalizing a segment of the personality from its entirety which permits the existence of dual or multiple personalities.

Ego That part of the personality which maintains contact with and evaluates reality, in order to establish or maintain a state of equilibrium within the self.

Elation An intense, unstable feeling of optimism, satisfaction or joy.

Emotion An intense, highly charged feeling.

Empathy A sustained quality of objective feeling with and for another without loss of one's personal perspective.

Euphoria An exaggerated sense of well-being.

Fear An emotional response to an immediate, known and exaggerated, external, definite or perceived danger which produces within the individual a feeling of disequilibrium.

Flight of ideas A constant, rapid, disconnected verbalization of thoughts.

Frustration A feeling state in which the individual experiences interference with the ability to achieve a specific goal, obtain satisfaction of a need or solve a problem.

Group A unit of society composed of two or more people in interaction.

Hallucination Is a false sensory perception for which there is no external stimuli.

Hostility A feeling state in which the individual, consciously or unconsciously, experiences a sense of helplessness and/or hopelessness associated with persons or objects toward whom negative attitudes or actions are directed.

Id The part of the mind which contains the primitive, instinctual impulses and urges and which operates on the pleasure principle.

Illusion A misinterpretation of a sensory perception.

Impulse The translation of thoughts into actions without regard to consequences.

Insight Self-understanding regarding motives, needs, wants and actions.

Instinct An innate, automatic reaction to a particular set of stimuli.

Mental mechanisms Are intrapsychic coping devices of ego defense existing outside of and beyond conscious awareness.

Mind A multisensory data bank which records, filters, processes and integrates all in-put.

Need An essential or requisite for the maintenance of life.

Negativism A generalized opposition to requests, demands or norms of others.

Neologism New words coined by the psychotic individual which are meaningful to the patient but meaningless to the listener.

Nursing care plan A written outline containing a systematized assessment and identification of the patient's problems, objectives for care and the methods or strategies for achieving the objectives.

Nursing diagnosis A summary statement or judgment made by the nurse about the data gathered during the assessment process.

Observation Is a deliberate, planned and systematized process of obtaining objective and subjective data.

Obsession Preoccupation with a persistent, repetitive thought.

Panic An acute, intense and overwhelming feeling of anxiety which results in a disorganization of various aspects of the personality.

Perception The recognition and interpretation of sensations.

Process A logical step by step progression of operations directed toward specific expected outcomes.

Psychogenic A term used to indicate that the pathological condition originates within the mind.

Rapport A feeling state of mutual sharing, openness and receptivity between individuals.

Relationship The existence of a connection or association between people.

Stress A real or perceived pressure that produces physiological and psychological change within the organism.

Superego That part of the personality which defines the value system under which the individual operates and acts as a censoring agent for all behavioral operations.

Sympathy A momentary feeling engendered within the nurse which evokes an immediate interventive response to alleviate the distress.

Therapeutic use of self The constructive use of the total personality of the nurse in a way which brings about a positive change for the patient.

Unconscious That part of the mind which records and stores all knowledge, feelings and experiences. Under ordinary circumstances this material is not readily accessible for recall to the conscious mind.

index

m

n

o